# Simply Kalorik Maxx Air Fryer Cookbook

*50 Effortless and Tasty Recipes to Enjoy the Crispness of Your Air Fryer Meals*

**Air Fryer Lab**

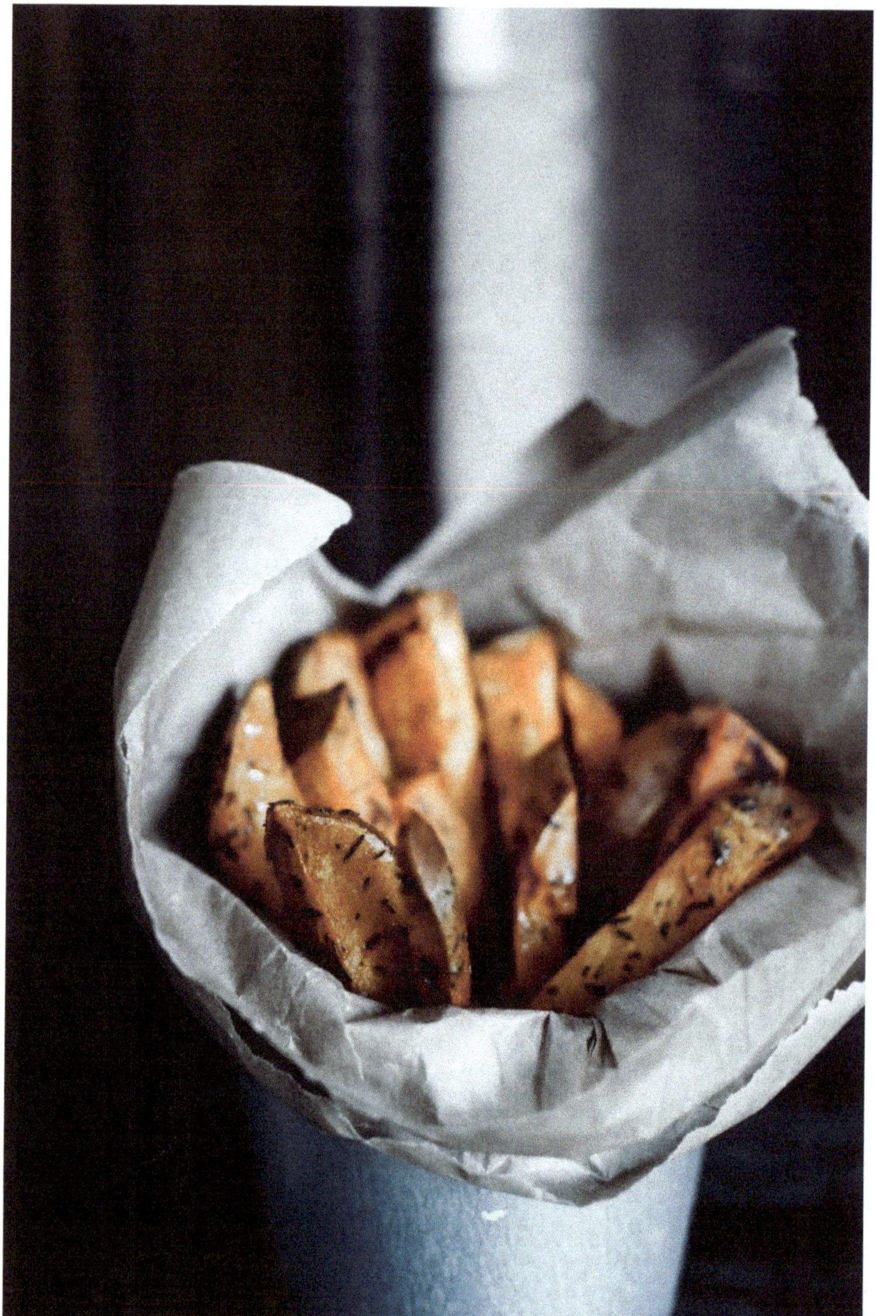

# Table of Content

# INTRODUCTION

Kalorik Maxx Air Fryer Oven is the newest addition to the Kalorik line. The Maxx Air Fryer is a convection oven, a toaster oven, and a multi-cooker rolled into one unit. It is the perfect kitchen tool for any home cook.

The Kalorik Maxx Air Fryer Oven features an innovative design that allows users to simultaneously bake, roast, sauté and fry without using any oil. It is ideal for year-round healthy cooking with the ability to perfectly crisp, cook and brown foods without added fat or oil.

The Kalorik Maxx Air Fryer Oven has a sleek and compact design which takes up little counter space. It can replace a conventional oven, toaster oven, infrared oven and multi-cooker making it ideal for those who are looking to make their kitchen clutter free.

Kalorik Maxx Air Fryer Oven is a very useful kitchen appliance that can utilize both convection oven and air frying capabilities. With it you can enjoy a delicious home-cooked meal even on a cold, windy day outside! And still, make your home warm and cozy.

The cookbook covers everything you may need to know about the Kalorik Maxx Air Fryer Oven. It can be used for double cooking, both for air frying and conventional cooking. Note that you should not mix convection and air frying modes! Conventional cooking is not recommended with Kalorik Maxx Air Fryer Oven except in some recipes where low fat or low-calorie dishes are desired.

With Kalorik Maxx Air Fryer Oven, you can enjoy the convenience of reheating your favorite TV dinner "on the fly". You can even set the temperature of your air frying and leave it unattended to cook your food in any required manner. Also, you can use the machine to make casseroles and other large meals because without a doubt it is a multi-purpose appliance.

The Kalorik Maxx Air Fryer Oven has several advantages:

- It cooks everything in about 10 minutes with less oil and shortening than conventional ovens or grills.
- It heats up your kitchen in no time by using radiant heating, which is much safer than using open flames.
- Because there are no hot parts inside the machine, it is safe for anyone to use.
- It utilizes convective heating, which will cook foods more evenly and faster. Unlike conventional ovens that cook foods with direct heat from the bottom, convection is a circulating current of air and uses electromagnetic waves to speed up cooking eliminating hot spots.
- It is easy to clean since there are no special cleaning tools required to open the top of the machine. It comes with an air cleaning system that automatically cleans all parts of the machine in about three minutes for a sparkling clean model.
- It utilizes a 3-in-1 function that can be used both as a convection oven and as an air fryer, so you can make dishes like fries, casseroles and popcorn.

The recipes in this cookbook are ideal for those who are fans of seafood, chicken, steak and pork because they have been prepared especially for Kalorik Maxx Air Fryer Oven. The recipes will make your mouth water and they are easy to cook. The cookbook is designed to make it easy for you to prepare delicious meals in a short time.

We hope you enjoy your Kalorik Maxx Air Fryer Oven while using this cookbook as a guide! We encourage creative cooks to add their own special touches, tastes and aromas.

Each recipe in this guide are cooked from start to finish in the Maxx Air Fryer.

The recipes in this guide were tested with the Kalorik Maxx Air Fryer Oven to ensure that the cooking times and temperatures used are accurate.  Let's get started!

# Appetizer and Snacks

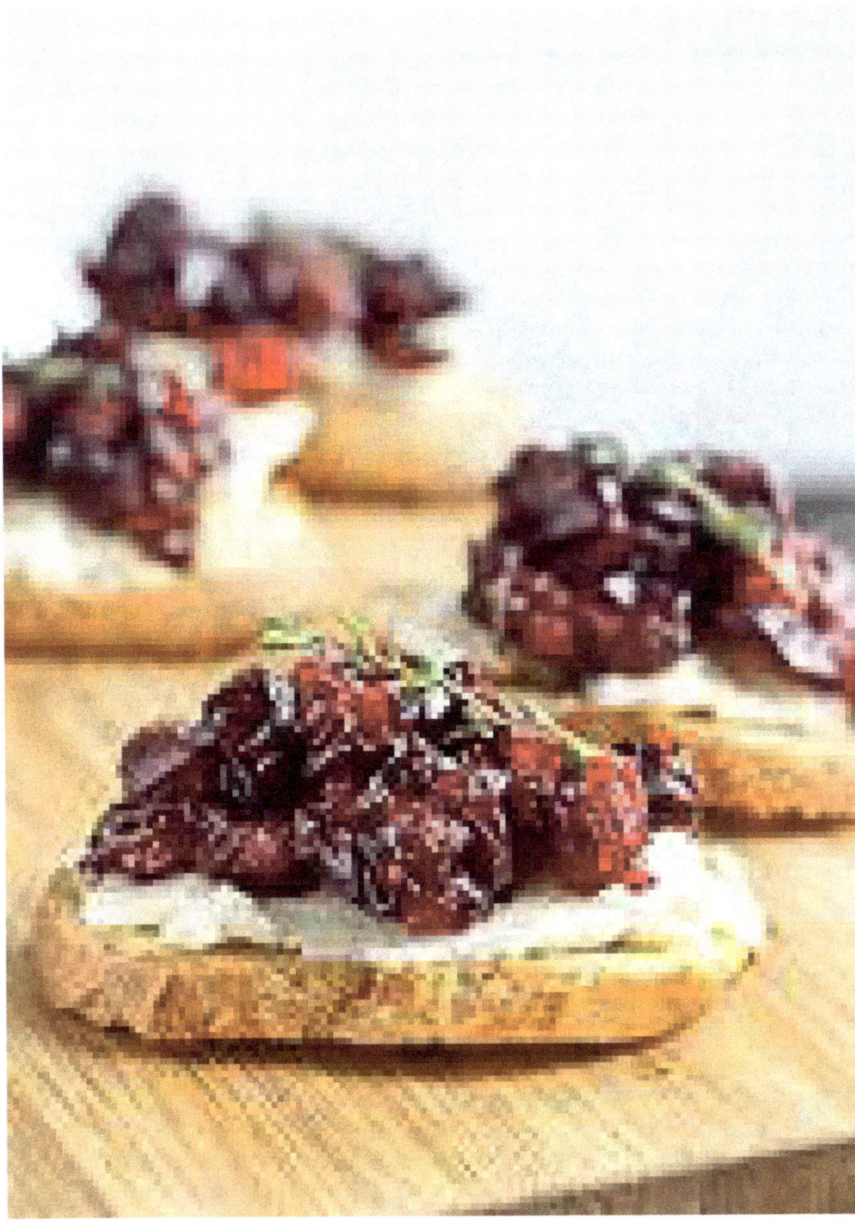

# Cheese Stuffed Jalapenos

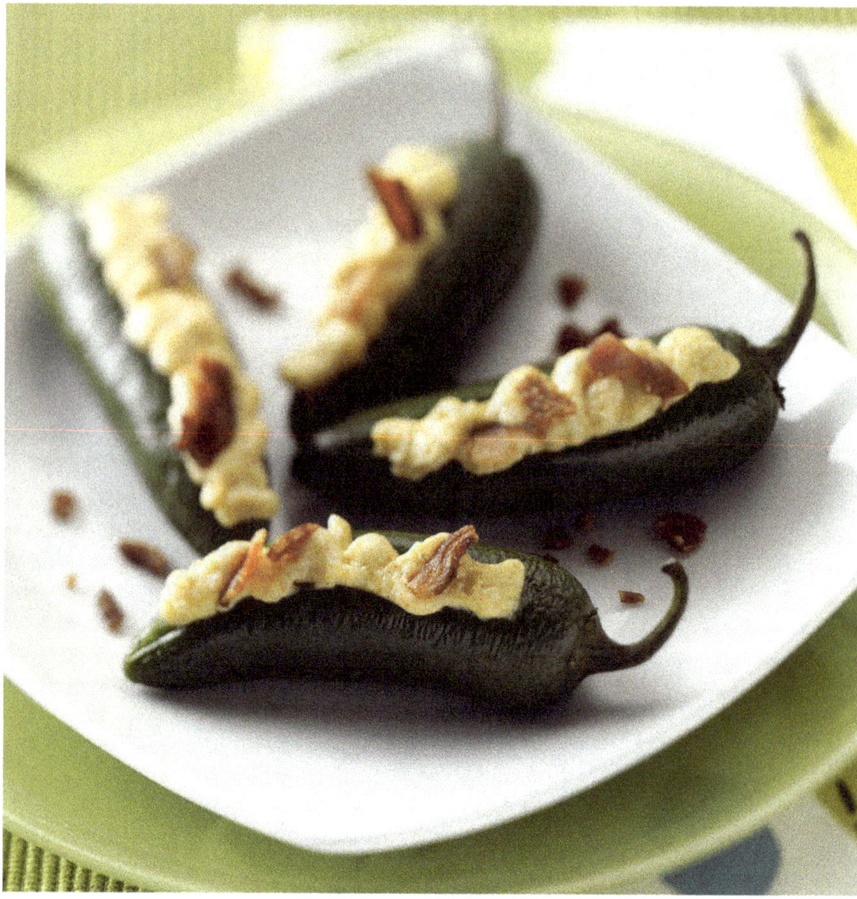

Preparation Time: 10 minutes

Cooking Time: 25 minutes

Servings: 4

**Ingredients:**

- 10jalapeno peppers, halved, remove seeds & membranes
- 1 tsp onion powder
- 1 tsp garlic powder

- 1 oz cheddar cheese, shredded
- 6oz cream cheese

**Directions:**

1. Spray cooking pan with cooking spray and set aside.
2. In a small bowl, mix together cream cheese, garlic powder, and onion powder.
3. Stuff cream cheese mixture into each jalapeno halves.
4. Place jalapeno halves onto the prepared cooking pan and top with shredded cheddar cheese.
5. Select bake mode and set the omni to 350 F for 25 minutes once the oven beeps, place the cooking pan into the oven.
6. Serve and enjoy.

**Nutrition:** Calories 196 Fat 17.7 g Carbohydrates 4.8 g Sugar 1.7 g Protein 5.7 g Cholesterol 54 mg

## Ranch Chickpeas

Preparation Time: 10 minutes

Cooking Time: 12 minutes

Servings: 12

**Ingredients:**

- 15oz can chickpeas, rinsed, drained, and pat dry
- 2tbsp ranch seasoning
- 1 tsp olive oil

**Directions:**

1 Line cooking pan with parchment paper and set aside.
2 In a mixing bowl, toss chickpeas with ranch seasoning and oil.
3 Spread chickpeas onto the prepared cooking pan.
4 Place cooking pan into the oven and select air fry mode set omni to the 380 F for 12 minutes. Stir chickpeas twice.
5 Serve and enjoy.

**Nutrition:** Calories 51 Fat 0.8 g Carbohydrates 8 g Sugar 0 g Protein 1.8 g Cholesterol 0 mg

## Cauliflower Hummus

Preparation Time: 10 minutes

Cooking Time: 35 minutes

Servings: 8

**Ingredients:**

- 1 cauliflower head, cut into florets
- 3tbsp olive oil
- 1/2 tsp ground cumin
- 1 tsp garlic, chopped
- tbsp fresh lemon juice
- 1/3 cup tahini
- Pepper
- Salt

**Directions:**

1 Spray cooking pan with cooking spray.
2 Spread cauliflower florets onto the prepared cooking pan.
3 Select bake mode and set the omni to 400 F for 35 minutes once the oven beeps, place the cooking pan into the oven. Turn cauliflower florets halfway through.
4 Transfer cauliflower florets into the food processor along with remaining ingredients and process until smooth.
5 Serve and enjoy.

**Nutrition:** Calories 115 Fat 10.7 g Carbohydrates 4.2 g Sugar 0.9 g Protein 2.4 g Cholesterol 0 mg

# Easy Roasted Brussels Sprouts

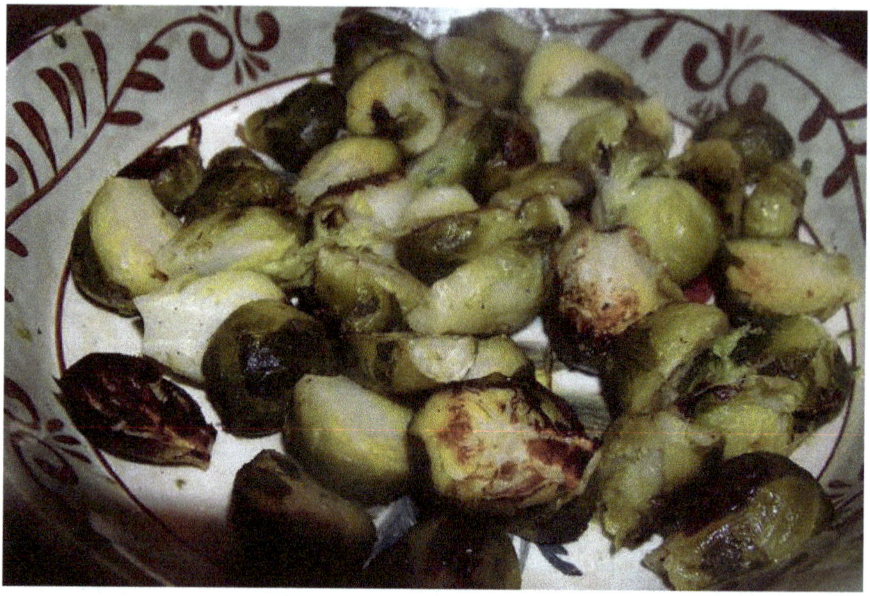

Preparation Time: 10 minutes

Cooking Time: 35 minutes

Servings: 6

**Ingredients:**

- 2cups Brussels sprouts, halved
- 1/4 tsp garlic powder
- 1/4 cup olive oil
- 1/4 tsp cayenne pepper
- 1/4 tsp salt

**Directions:**

1 Add all ingredients into the large bowl and toss well.
2 Transfer Brussels sprouts on a cooking pan.

3 Select bake mode and set the omni to 400 F for 35 minutes once the oven beeps, place the cooking pan into the oven. Turn halfway through.
4 Serve and enjoy.

**Nutrition:** Calories 85 Fat 8.5 g Carbohydrates 2.8 g Sugar 0.7 g Protein 1 g Cholesterol 0 mg

## Air Fried Cauliflower Florets

Preparation Time: 10 minutes

Cooking Time: 15 minutes

Servings: 4

**Ingredients:**

- 1 medium cauliflower head, cut into florets
- 1/2 tsp old bay seasoning
- 1/4 tsp paprika
- 1 tbsp garlic, minced
- 3tbsp olive oil
- Pepper
- Salt

**Directions:**

1 In a large bowl, toss cauliflower with remaining ingredients.

2 Spread cauliflower florets onto the cooking pan.

3 Place cooking pan into the oven and select air fry mode set omni to the 400 F for 15 minutes. Stir twice.

4 Serve and enjoy.

**Nutrition:** Calories 130 Fat 10.7 g Carbohydrates 8.4 g Sugar 3.5 g Protein 3 g Cholesterol 0 mg

## Herb Mushrooms

Preparation Time: 10 minutes

Cooking Time: 14 minutes

Servings: 4

**Ingredients:**

- 1 lb mushrooms
- 1/2 tsp ground coriander
- 1 tsp rosemary, chopped
- 1 tbsp basil, minced
- 1 garlic clove, minced
- 1/2 tbsp vinegar
- Pepper
- Salt

**Directions:**

1 Add all ingredients into the large bowl and toss well.

2 Spread mushrooms onto the cooking pan.

3 Place cooking pan into the oven and select air fry mode set omni to the 350 F for 14 minutes. Stir halfway through.

4 Serve and enjoy.

**Nutrition:** Calories 27 Fat 0.4 g Carbohydrates 4.2 g Sugar 2 g Protein 3.6 g Cholesterol 0 mg

# Cinnamon Sweet Potato Bites

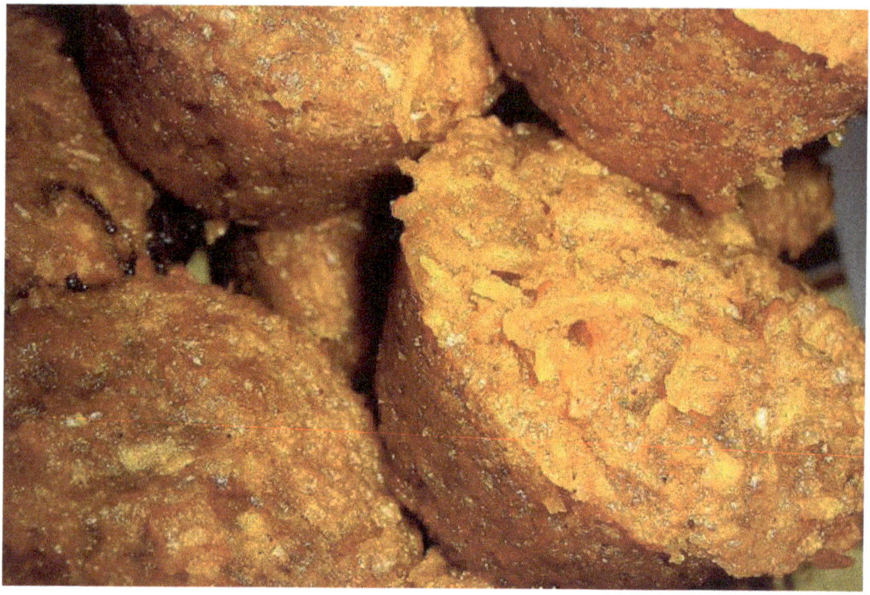

Preparation Time: 10 minutes

Cooking Time: 15 minutes

Servings: 2

**Ingredients:**

- 2sweet potato, diced into 1-inch cubes
- 1 1/2 tsp cinnamon
- 2tbsp olive oil
- 2tbsp honey
- 1 tsp red chili flakes
- 1/2 cup fresh parsley, chopped

**Directions:**

1 Add all ingredients into the bowl and toss well.

2 Spread sweet potato cubes onto the cooking pan.

3 Place cooking pan into the oven and select air fry mode set omni to the 350 F for 15 minutes. Stir halfway through.
4 Serve and enjoy.

**Nutrition:** Calories 297 Fat 14.3 g Carbohydrates 43.2 g Sugar 24.8 g Protein 2.9 g Cholesterol 0 mg

# Breakfast and Dessert

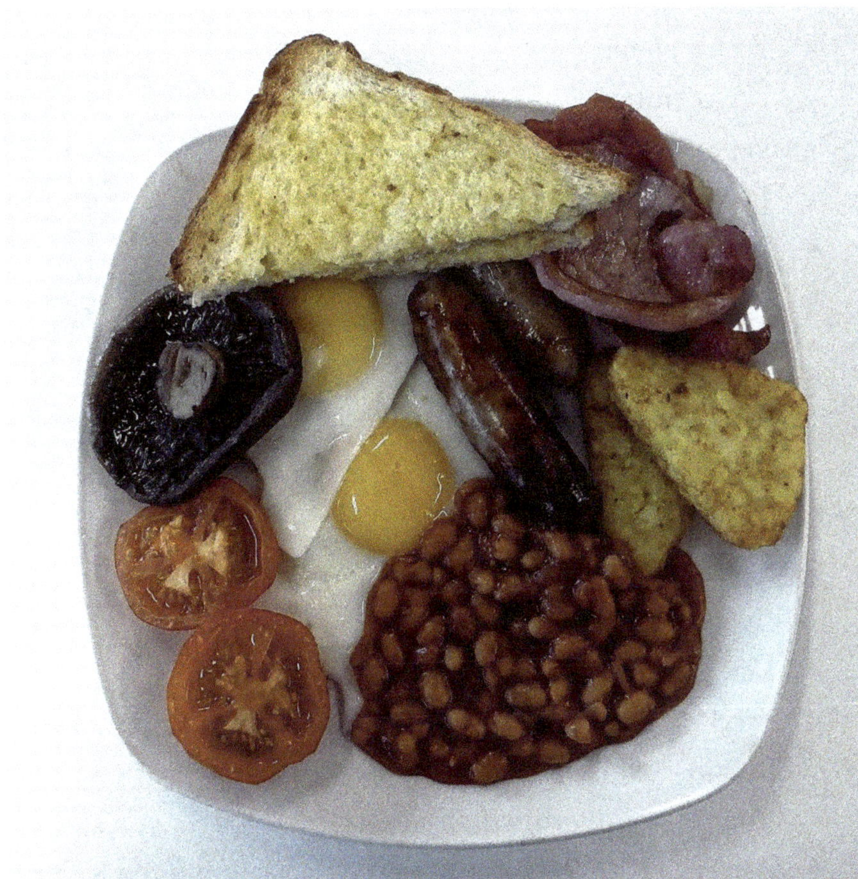

## Baked Apple

Preparation time: 5 minutes

Cooking time: 20 minutes

Servings: 4

**Ingredients:**

- ¼ cup water
- ¼ tsp. nutmeg
- ¼ tsp. cinnamon
- 1 ½ tsp. melted ghee
- 2tbsp. raisins
- 2tbsp. chopped walnuts
- 1 medium apple

**Directions**

1 Preparing the Ingredients. Preheat your air fryer to 350 degrees Fahrenheit.
2 Slice an apple in half and discard some of the flesh from the center.
3 Place into frying pan.
4 Mix remaining ingredients together except water. Spoon mixture to the middle of apple halves.
5 Pour water overfilled apples.
6 Air Frying. Place pan with apple halves into the Kalorik Maxx air fryer, bake 20 minutes.

**Nutrition:** Calories 199 Fat 9g Protein 1g Sugar 3g

## Cinnamon Fried Bananas

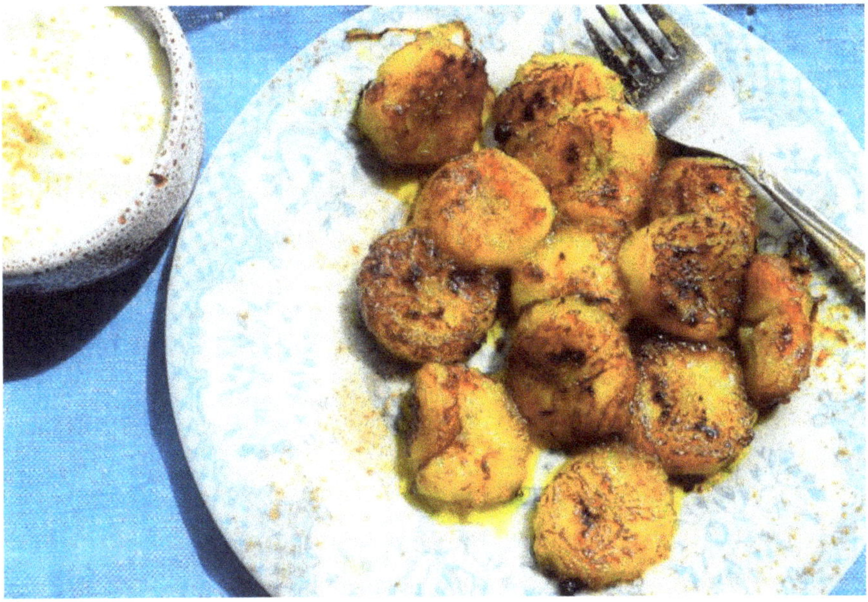

Preparation time: 5 minutes

Cooking time: 10 minutes

Servings: 2-3

**Ingredients:**

- 1 cup panko breadcrumbs
- 3tbsp. cinnamon
- ½ cup almond flour
- 3egg whites
- 8ripe bananas
- 3tbsp. vegan coconut oil

**Directions**

1 Preparing the Ingredients. Heat coconut oil and add breadcrumbs. Mix around 2-3 minutes until golden. Pour into bowl.

2 Peel and cut bananas in half. Roll each bananas half into flour, eggs, and crumb mixture.

3 Air Frying. Place into the Kalorik Maxx air fryer. Cook 10 minutes at 280 degrees Fahrenheit.

4 A great addition to a healthy banana split!

**Nutrition:** Calories 219 Fat 10g Protein 3g Sugar 5g

# Awesome Chinese Doughnuts

Preparation time: 10 minutes

Cooking time: 8 minutes

Servings: 8

**Ingredients:**

- 1 tbsp. baking powder
- 1tbsps. coconut oil
- ¾ cup of coconut milk
- 6tsps. sugar
- 2cup all-purpose flour
- ½ tsp. sea salt

**Directions**

1 Preheat the air fryer to 350 degrees Fahrenheit.
2 Mix baking powder, flour, sugar, and salt in a bowl.
3 Add coconut oil and mix well. Add coconut milk and mix until well combined.
4 Knead dough for 3-4 minutes.
5 Roll dough half inch thick and using cookie cutter cut doughnuts.
6 Place doughnuts in cake pan and brush with oil. Place cake pan in air fryer basket and air fry doughnuts for 5 minutes. Turn doughnuts to other side and air fry for 3 minutes more.
7 Serve and enjoy.

**Nutrition:** Calories 259 Fat 15.9g Carbohydrates 27g Protein 3.8g

## Crispy Bananas

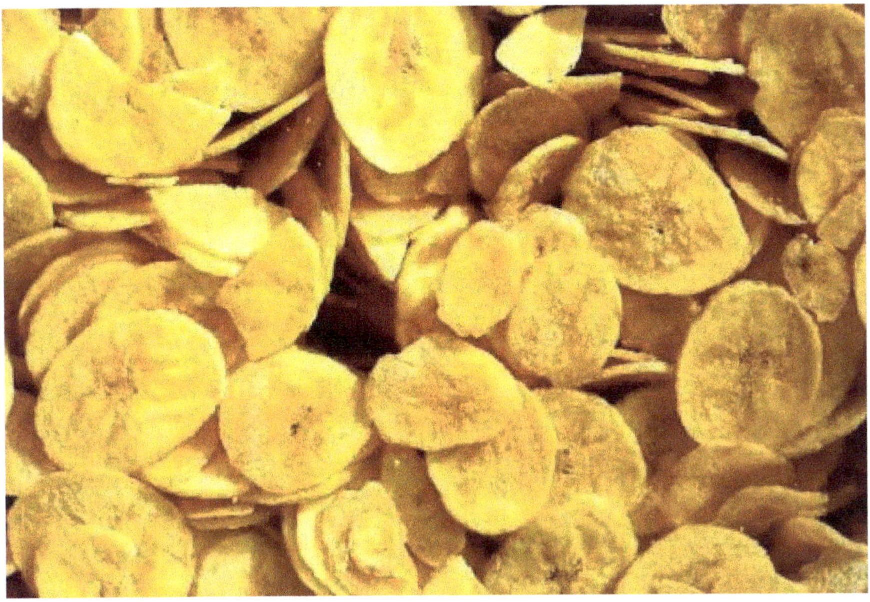

Preparation time: 10 minutes

Cooking time: 10 minutes

Servings: 4

**Ingredients:**

- 4 sliced ripe bananas
- 1 egg
- ½ cup breadcrumbs
- 1 ½ tbsps. cinnamon sugar
- 1 tbsp. almond meal
- 1 ½ tbsps. coconut oil
- 1 tbsp. crushed cashew
- ¼ cup corn flour

**Directions**

1. Set the pan on fire to heat the coconut oil over medium heat and add breadcrumbs in the pan and stir for 3-4 minutes.
2. Remove pan from heat and transfer breadcrumbs in a bowl.
3. Add almond meal and crush cashew in breadcrumbs and mix well.
4. Dip banana half in corn flour then in egg and finally coat with breadcrumbs.
5. Place coated banana in air fryer basket. Sprinkle with Cinnamon Sugar.
6. Air fry at 350 degrees Fahrenheit/ 176 degrees Celsius for 10 minutes.
7. Serve and enjoy.

**Nutrition:** Calories 282 Fat 9g Carbohydrates 46g Protein 5g

# Air Fried Banana and Walnuts Muffins

Preparation time: 10 minutes

Cooking time: 10 minutes

Servings: 2

**Ingredients:**

- ¼ cup flour
- ½ tsp. baking powder
- ¼ cup mashed banana
- ¼ cup butter
- 1 tbsp. chopped walnuts
- ¼ cup oats

**Directions**

1 Spray four muffin molds with cooking spray and set aside.

2 In a bowl, mix together mashed bananas, walnuts, sugar, and butter.

3 In another bowl, mix oat flour, and baking powder.

4 Combine the flour mixture to the banana mixture.

5 Pour batter into prepared muffin mold.

6 Place in air fryer basket and cook at 320 degrees Fahrenheit/ 160 degrees Celsius for 10 minutes.

7 Remove muffins from air fryer and allow to cool completely.

8 Serve and enjoy.

**Nutrition:** Calories 192 Fat 12.3g Carbohydrates 19.4g Protein 1.9g

# Pears and espresso cream

Preparation time: 10 minutes

cooking time:30 minutes

servings: 4

**Ingredients:**

- `4 pears, halved and cored
- `2 tbsp. Water
- `2 tbsp. Lemon juice
- `1 tbsp. Sugar
- `2 tbsp. Butter
- `For the cream:
- `1 cup whipping cream
- `2 tbsp. Espresso, cold
- `1 cup mascarpone
- `1/3 cup sugar

**Directions:**

1 In a bowl mix pears halves with lemon juice, 1 tbsp. Sugar, butter and water, toss well, transfer them to your air fryer and cook at 360 °f for 30 minutes

2 Meanwhile in a bowl, mix whipping cream with mascarpone, ⅓ cup sugar and espresso, whisk really well and keep in the fridge until pears are done.

3 Divide pears on plates, top with espresso cream and serve them

**Nutrition:** Calories 211 fats: 5 g carbs 8 g proteins 7 g

## Nutty Mix

Preparation time: 5 minutes

Cooking time: 4 minutes

Servings: 6

**Ingredients:**

- 2cup mix nuts
- 1 tsp. ground cumin
- 1 tsp. chili powder
- 1 tbsp. melted butter
- 1 tsp. salt
- 1 tsp. pepper

**Directions**

1. Set all ingredients in a large bowl and toss until well coated.
2. Preheat the air fryer at 350 degrees Fahrenheit for 5 minutes.
3. Add mix nuts in air fryer basket and air fry for 4 minutes. Shake basket halfway through.
4. Serve and enjoy.

**Nutrition:** Calories 316 Fat 29g Carbohydrates 11.3g Protein 7.6g

# Vanilla Spiced Soufflé

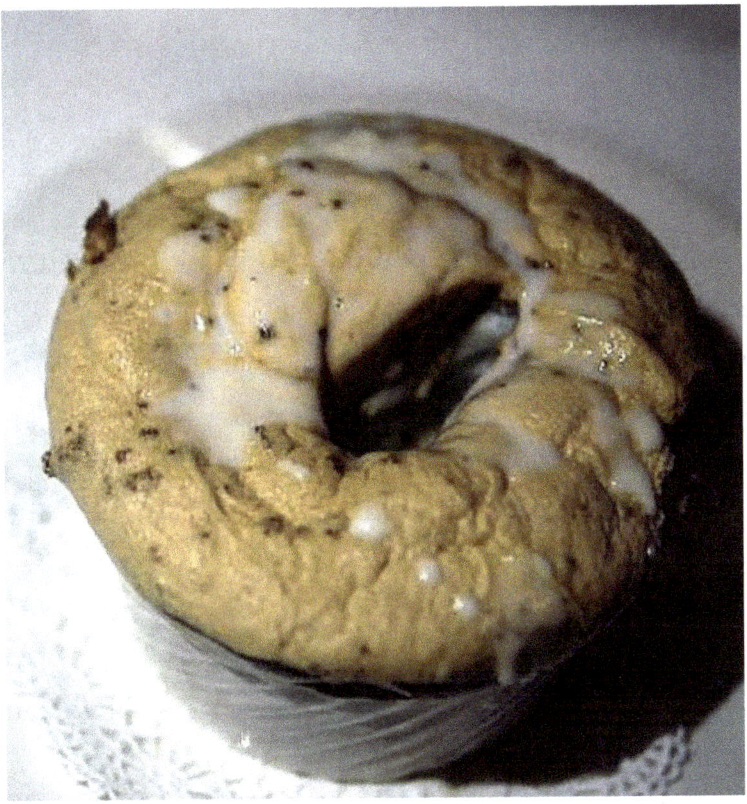

Preparation time: 20 minutes

Cooking time: 32 minutes

Servings: 6

**Ingredients:**

- ¼ cup all-purpose flour
- 1 cup whole milk
- 2tsps. vanilla extract
- 1 tsp. cream of tartar
- 1 vanilla bean

- 4egg yolks
- 1-oz. sugar
- ¼ cup softened butter
- ¼ cup sugar
- 5egg whites

**Directions**

1. Combine flour and butter in a bowl until the mixture becomes a smooth paste.
2. Set the pan over medium flame to heat the milk. Add sugar and stir until dissolved.
3. Mix in the vanilla bean and bring to a boil.
4. Beat the mixture using a wire whisk as you add the butter and flour mixture.
5. Lower the heat to simmer until thick. Discard the vanilla bean. Turn off the heat.
6. Place them on an ice bath and allow to cool for 10 minutes.
7. Grease 6 ramekins with butter. Sprinkle each with a bit of sugar.
8. Beat the egg yolks in a bowl. Add the vanilla extract and milk mixture. Mix until combined.
9. Whisk together the tartar cream, egg whites, and sugar until it forms medium stiff peaks.
10. Gradually fold egg whites into the soufflé base. Transfer the mixture to the ramekins.
11. Put 3 ramekins in the cooking basket at a time. Cook for 16 minutes at 330 degrees Fahrenheit. Move to a wire rack for cooling and cook the rest.

12. Sprinkle powdered sugar on top and drizzle with chocolate sauce before serving.

**Nutrition:** Calories 215 Fat 12.2g Carbohydrates 18.98g Protein 6.66g

# Chocolate Cup Cakes

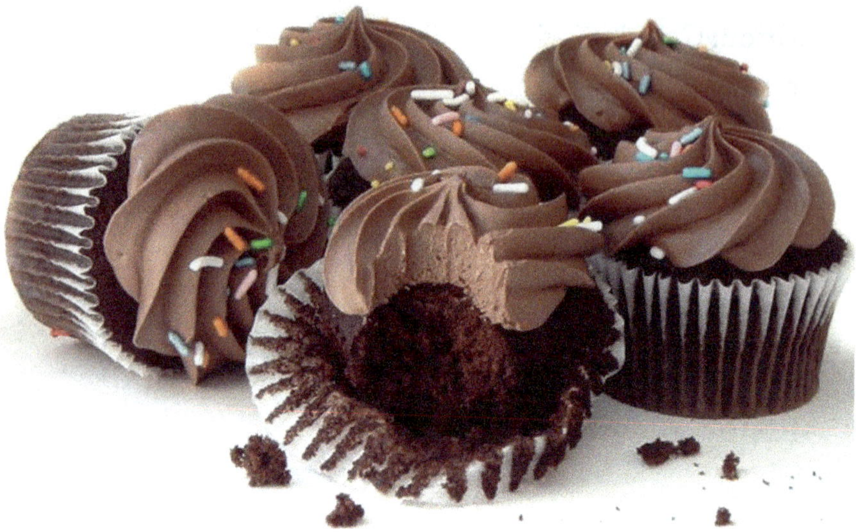

Preparation time: 5 minutes

Cooking time: 12 minutes

Servings: 6

**Ingredients:**

- 3eggs
- ¼ cup caster sugar
- ¼ cup cocoa powder
- 1 tsp. baking powder
- 1 cup milk
- ¼ tsp. vanilla essence
- 2cup all-purpose flour
- 4tbsps. butter

**Directions**

1. Preheat your Air Fryer to a temperature of 400 degrees Fahrenheit (200 degrees Celsius).
2. Beat eggs with sugar in a bowl until creamy.
3. Add butter and beat again for 1-2 minutes.
4. Now add flour, cocoa powder, milk, baking powder, and vanilla essence, mix with a spatula.
5. Fill ¾ of muffin tins with the mixture and place them into Air Fryer basket.
6. Let cook for 12 minutes.
7. Serve!

**Nutrition:** Calories 289 Fat 11.5g Carbohydrates 38.94g Protein 8.72g

## Air Baked Cheesecake

Preparation time: 20 minutes

Cooking time: 20 minutes

Servings: 8-12

**Ingredients:**

Crust

- 1/2 cup dates, chopped, soaked in water for at least 15 min., soaking liquid reserved
- 1/2 cup walnuts
- 1 cup quick oats

Filling

- 1/2 cup vanilla almond milk
- 1/4 cup coconut palm sugar
- 1/2 cup coconut flour
- 1 cup cashews, soaked in water for at least 2 hours
- 1 tsp. vanilla extract
- 2tbsp. lemon juice
- 1 to 2 tsp. grated lemon zest
- 1/2 cup fresh berries or 6 figs, sliced
- 1 tbsp. arrowroot powder

**Directions:**

1. Make the crust: in a food processor, process together all the crust ingredients until smooth and press the mixture into the bottom of a spring form pan.

2. Make the filling: add cashews along with soaking liquid to a blender and process until very smooth; add milk, palm sugar, coconut flour, lemon juice, lemon zest, and vanilla and blend until well combined; add arrowroot and continue blending until mixed and pour into the crust. Smooth the top and cover the spring form pan with foil.
3. Place the pan in your air fry toaster oven and bake at 375 degrees Fahrenheit for 20 minutes.
4. Carefully remove the pan from the fryer and remove the foil; let the cake cool completely and top with fruit to serve.

**Nutrition:** Calories 423 Fat 3.1g Carbohydrates 33.5g Protein 1.2g

# Soup and Stews

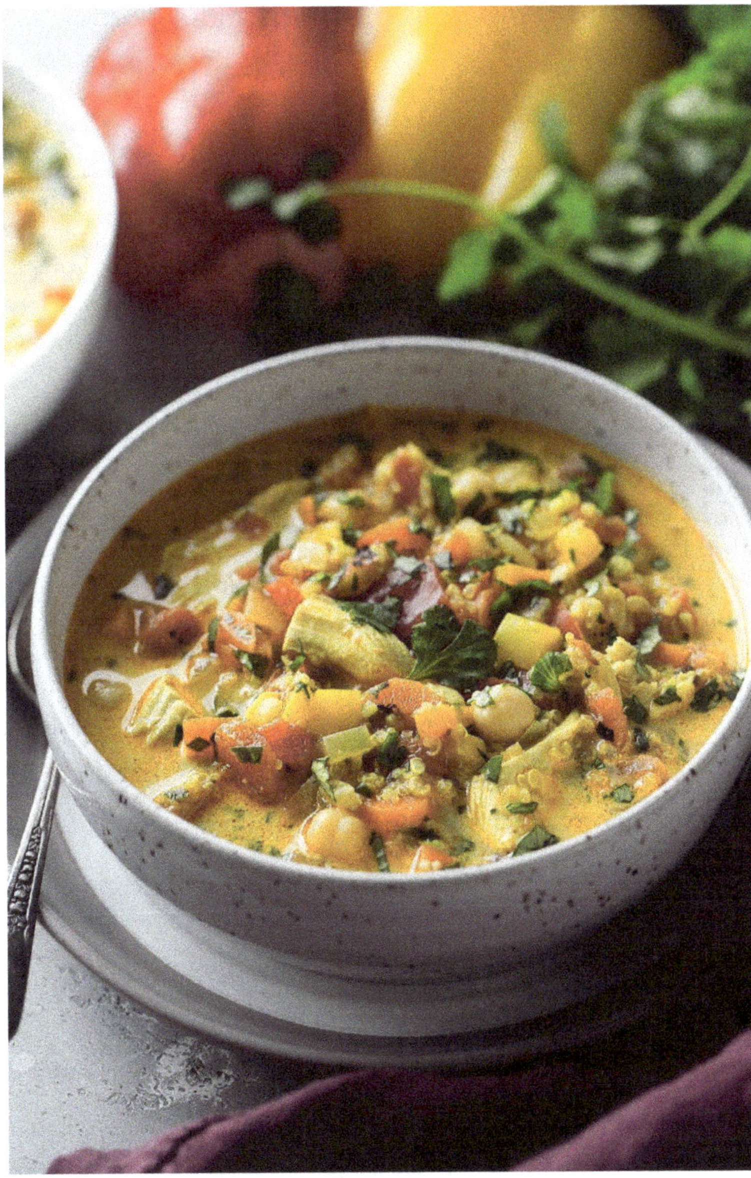

## Air Fried Carrots, Yellow Squash & Zucchini

Preparation Time: 5 minutes

Cooking time: 35 minutes

Servings: 4

**Ingredients:**

- 1 tbsp. chopped tarragon leaves
- ½ tsp. white pepper
- 1 tsp. salt
- 1 pound yellow squash
- 1 pound zucchini
- 6 tsp. olive oil
- ½ pound carrots

**Directions:**

1. Stem and root the end of squash and zucchini and cut in ¾-inch half-moons. Peel and cut carrots into 1-inch cubes Combine carrot cubes with 2 teaspoons of olive oil, tossing to combine.
2. Pour into the Chefman Air Fryer Oven basket, set temperature to 400°F, and set time to 5 minutes.
3. As carrots cook, drizzle remaining olive oil over squash and zucchini pieces, then season with pepper and salt. Toss well to coat.

4. Add squash and zucchini when the timer for carrots goes off. Cook 30 minutes, making sure to toss 2-3 times during the cooking process.
5. Once done, take out veggies and toss with tarragon. Serve up warm.

**Nutrition:** Calories: 122 Cal Total Fat: 9 g Saturated Fat: 0 g Cholesterol: 0 mg Sodium: 0 mg Total Carbs: 0 g Fiber: 0 g Sugar: 0 g Protein: 6 g

# Low Carb Taco Soup

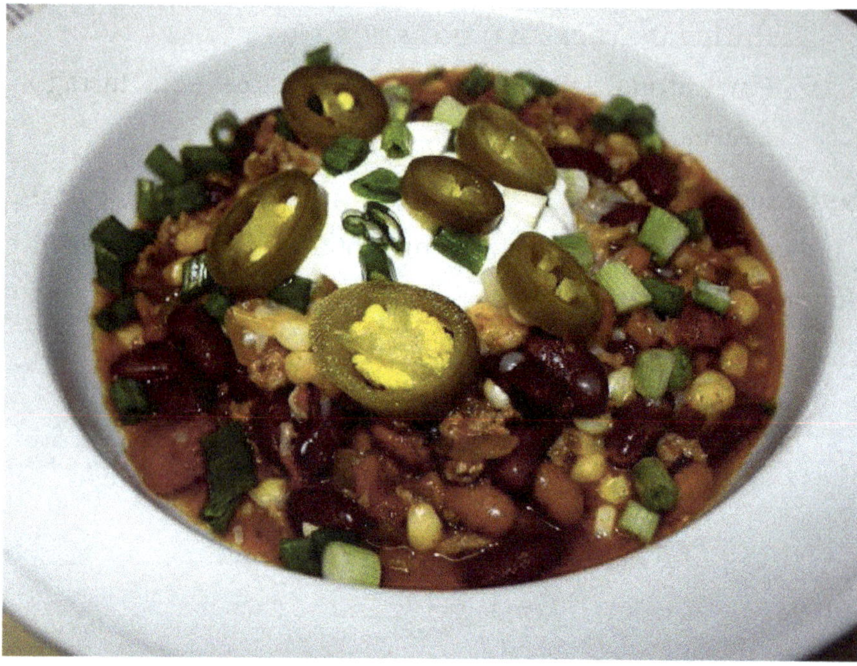

Preparation Time: 25 minutes

Cooking time: 20 minutes

Servings: 4

**Ingredients:**

- 1 tbsp. olive oil
- lbs. ground beef
- 1 onion, diced
- 1 bell pepper, diced
- tbsp. garlic, minced
- tbsp. cumin
- 1 tsp. paprika
- 1 tsp. salt

- 1 tsp. pepper
- 1 cup shredded cheese
- 1 tsp. Sriracha
- 14.5 oz. can tomato, diced
- oz. can green chilies
- cups beef broth
- tbsp. chili powder

**Directions**

1 In a pan that fits the air fryer oven, mix all the ingredients, toss, introduce in the fryer and cook at 380 degrees Fahrenheit for 20 minutes

2 Divide the stew into bowls and serve for lunch.

**Nutrition:** Calories 183 Fat 4g Fiber 2g Carbohydrates 4g Protein 12g

## Mexican Beef Soup

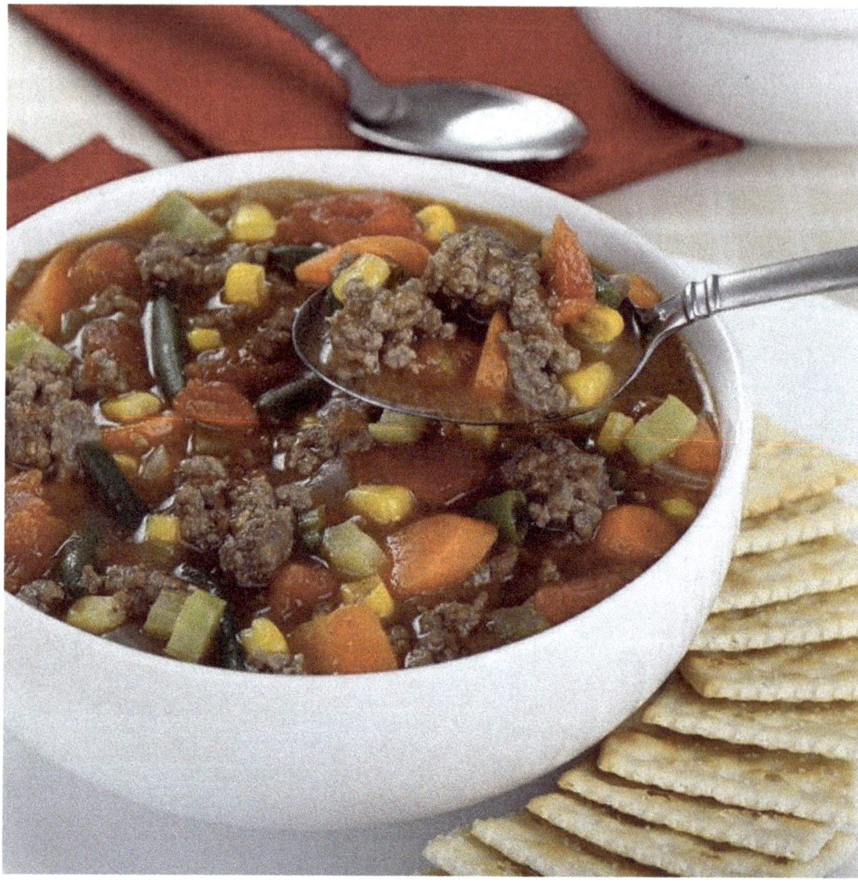

Preparation Time: 30 minutes

Cooking time: 25 minutes

Servings: 4

**Ingredients:**

- 1-pound beef stew meat
- 3/4-pound potatoes cut into 3/4-inch cubes
- cups frozen corn, thawed

- medium carrots, cut into 1/2-inch slices
- 1 medium onion, chopped
- garlic cloves, minced
- 1-1/2 tsp. dried oregano
- 1 tsp. ground cumin
- 1/2 tsp. salt
- 1/4 tsp. crushed red pepper flakes
- cups beef stock
- 1 can diced tomatoes and green chilies

**Directions**

1. In a baking dish that fits your air fryer oven, mix the turkey with the rest of the ingredients except the parsley, toss, introduce the dish in the fryer, bake at 380 degrees Fahrenheit for 25 minutes
2. Divide into bowls, sprinkle the parsley on top and serve.

**Nutrition:** Calories 250 Fat 11g Fiber 2g Carbohydrates 6g Protein 12g

## Zucchini and Cauliflower Stew

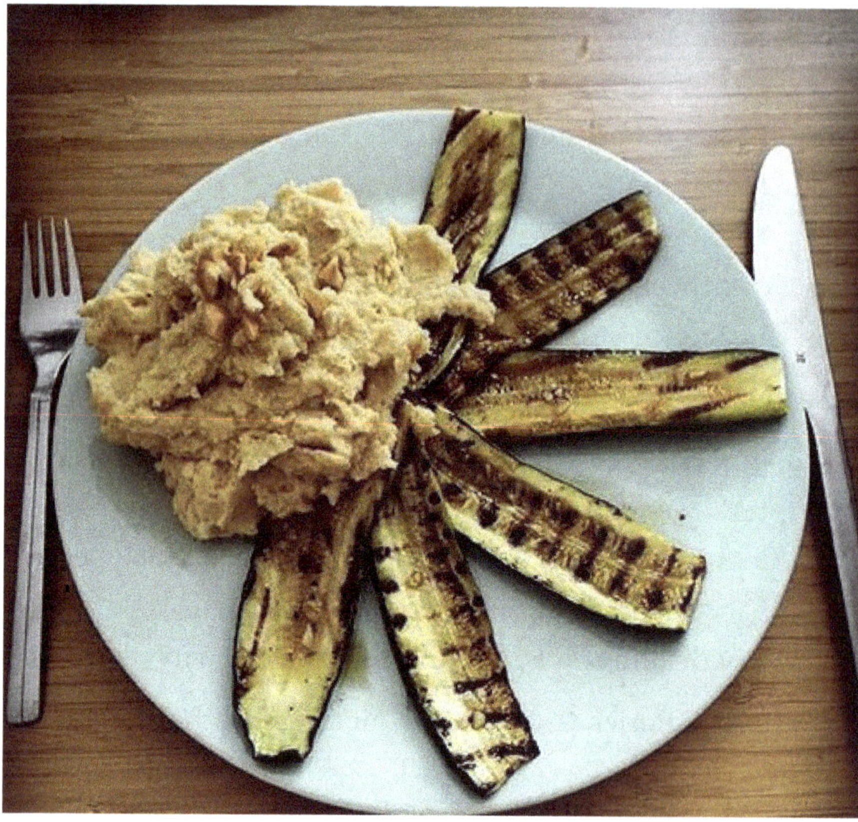

Preparation Time: 25 minutes

Cooking time: 20 minutes

Servings: 4

**Ingredients:**

- 1 cauliflower head, florets separated
- 1 ½ cups zucchinis; sliced
- 1 handful parsley leaves; chopped.
- ½ cup tomato puree
- green onions; chopped.

- 1 tbsp. balsamic vinegar
- 1 tbsp. olive oil
- Salt and black pepper to taste.

**Directions**

1. In a pan that fits your air fryer oven, mix the zucchinis with the rest of the ingredients except the parsley, toss, introduce the pan in the air fryer oven and cook at 380 degrees Fahrenheit for 20 minutes
2. Divide into bowls and serve for lunch with parsley sprinkled on top.

**Nutrition:** Calories 193 Fat 5g Fiber 2g Carbohydrates 4g Protein 7g

# Butternut Squash and Apple Soup

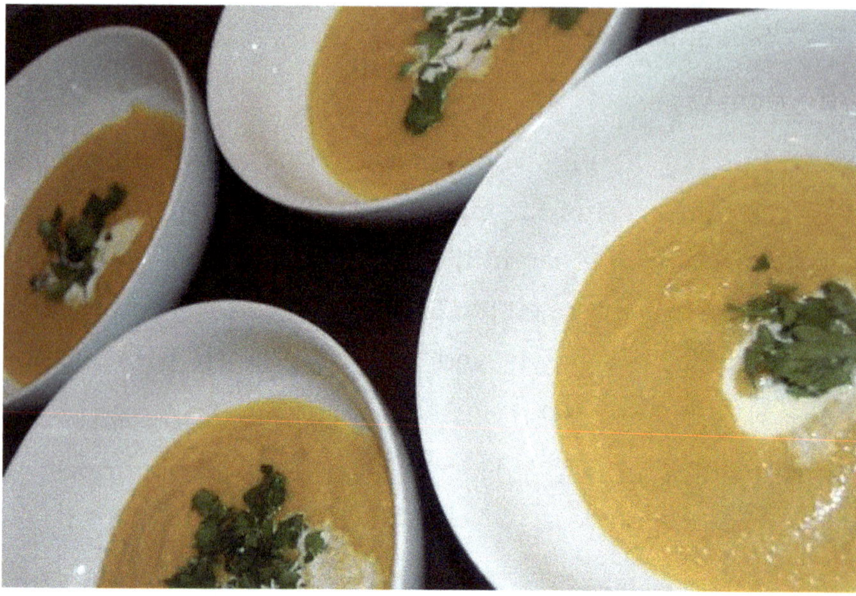

Preparation Time: 35 minutes

Cooking time: 30 minutes

Servings: 6

**Ingredients:**

- 2tbsp. olive oil
- 1 onion, chopped
- 1 tsp. dried sage
- 1/3 cup Cashew Milk
- ¼ tsp. salt
- ¼ tsp. pepper
- cloves garlic, minced
- 1 (2 pounds) butternut squash, seeded, and cut into 1-inch cubes

- 2apples, cored and diced into 1-inch chunks
- 1cups vegetable stock

**Directions**

1 Grease a baking dish that fits your air fryer oven with the butter, add all the ingredients in the pan and toss them.

2 Introduce the dish in the fryer, cook at 360 degrees Fahrenheit for 30 minutes, divide into bowls and serve

**Nutrition:** Calories 246 Fat 12g Fiber 2g Carbohydrates 6g Protein 12g

# Carrot Soup

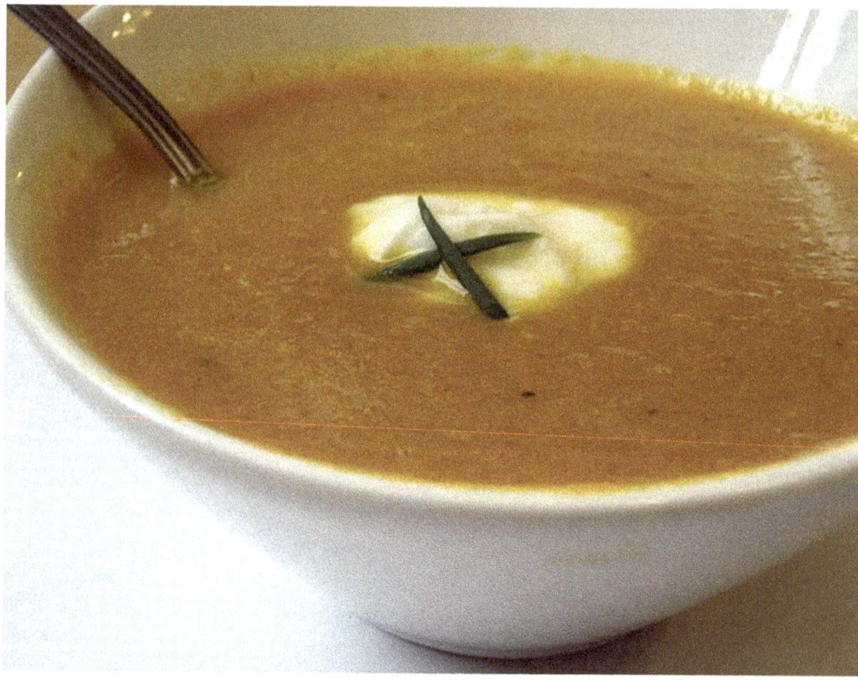

Preparation Time: 35 minutes

Cooking time: 30 minutes

Servings: 4

**Ingredients:**

- `1 tbsp. unsalted butter
- `1 tbsp. oil
- `1 onion, chopped
- `¼ tsp. kosher salt
- `¼ tsp. pepper
- `2 cups low-sodium chicken broth
- `13.5 oz. can unsweetened coconut milk

- `1 tbsp. Sriracha
- `1 clove garlic, minced
- `1 tbsp. minced ginger
- `1-pound carrots, chopped
- `1/4 tsp. brown sugar

**Directions**

1 In a pan that fits your air fryer oven, mix all the ingredients, toss, introduce in your air fryer oven and cook at 370 degrees Fahrenheit for 30 minutes

2 Divide into bowls and serve right away.

**Nutrition:** Calories 245 Fat 12g Fiber 2g Carbohydrates 5g Protein 14g

## Chicken Gnocchi Soup

Preparation Time: 10 minutes

Cooking time: 18 minutes

Servings: 3

**Ingredients:**

- `2 tbsp. butter
- `1 tbsp. olive oil
- `2 onions, diced
- `2 cloves garlic, minced
- `2 large carrots
- `1 cup spinach
- `1 16-ounce package potato gnocchi
- `3 tbsp. flour
- `4 cups water
- `1 tbsp. thyme leaves
- `1-pound chicken breast
- `½ tsp. salt
- `½ tsp. pepper
- `2 cups whole milk

**Directions**

1 Set the Air fryer oven to 375 degrees F for 5 minutes.

2 Put the garlic, onion, potato gnocchi in the cooking tray. Insert the cooking tray in the Oven when it displays "Add Food".

3. Remove from the oven when Cooking Time is complete. Put the butter in a wok and add the garlic mixture, black beans, tomato paste, water, salt and black pepper.
4. Sauté for about 3 minutes and stir in the sour and fresh creams. Secure the lid of the wok and cook for about 10 minutes on medium heat.
5. Puree the contents of the soup with an immersion blender and serve with nachos chips.

**Nutrition:** Calories 339 Fat 13.1g Carbohydrates 45g Protein 13.1g

## Chicken Noodle Soup

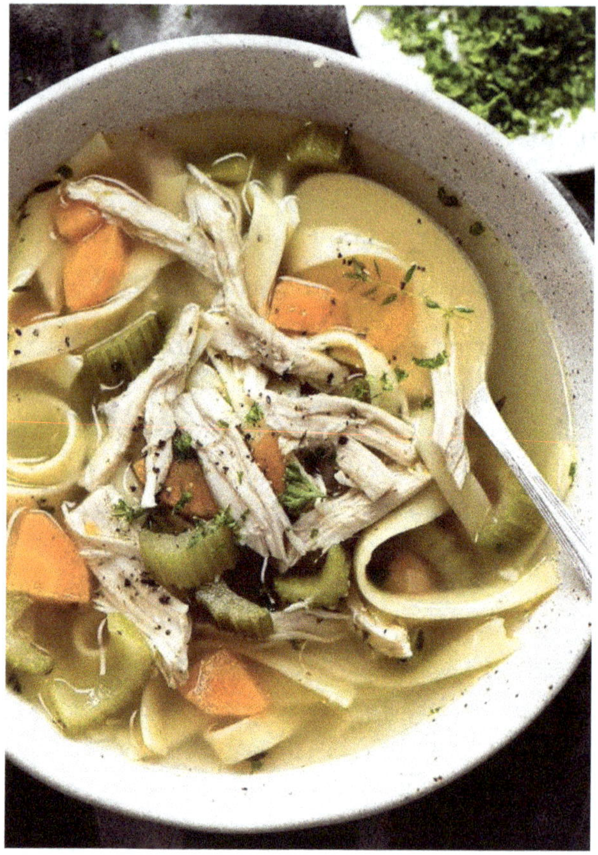

Preparation Time: 10 minutes

Cooking time: 20 minutes

Servings: 4

**Ingredients:**

- `1 tbsp. olive oil
- `1 onion, diced
- `3 cloves of garlic, minced
- `½ tbsp. pepper

- `4 oz. of extra-wide egg noodles
- `1/4 cup of minced flat-leaf parsley
- `5 carrots, sliced into 1/2-inch chunks
- `2 celery sticks, sliced into 1/2-inch pieces
- `1 whole 5-pound chicken giblets removed and discarded
- `2 tbsp. soy sauce
- `8 cups water
- `½ tbsp. salt

**Directions**

1 Cook onion in olive oil at Sauté for 2-3 minutes.

2 Add garlic, carrots and celery and sauté for 1 minute.

3 Add whole chicken, soy sauce, 2 teaspoon of salt and several turns of freshly ground pepper in a cooking stove for 20 minutes and remove.

4 Turn Kalorik Maxx to Sauté and let the chicken broth come to a boil.

5 Add egg noodles and let cook for about 5 minutes.

6 Once noodles are cooked, add shredded chicken and fresh parsley and serve.

**Nutrition:** Calories 344 Fat 16.7g Carbohydrates 44.1g Protein 8.3g

## Vegetable Wild Rice Soup

Preparation Time: 10 minutes

Cooking time: 15 minutes

Servings: 4

**Ingredients:**

- `6 cups reduced-sodium vegetable broth
- `2 cans (14-1/2 ounces each) fire-roasted diced tomatoes, undrained
- `2 celery ribs, sliced
- `2 medium carrots, chopped
- `1-3/4 cups baby Portobello mushrooms, sliced
- `1 onion, chopped
- `1 parsnip, peeled and chopped
- `1 sweet potato, peeled and cubed
- `1 green pepper, chopped
- `1 cup uncooked wild rice
- `2 garlic cloves, minced
- `3/4 tsp. salt
- `1/4 tsp. pepper
- `2 bay leaves
- `2 fresh thyme sprigs

**Directions**

1 Set the Air fryer oven to 375 degrees Fahrenheit for 5 minutes.

2 Put all ingredients in the cooking tray.

3. Insert the cooking tray in the oven.
4. Remove from the oven when Cooking Time is complete. Put the butter in a wok and add the garlic mixture, white beans, tomato paste, water, salt and white pepper.
5. Sauté for about 3 minutes and stir in the fresh cream. Secure the lid of the wok and cook for about 12 minutes on medium heat.

**Nutrition:** Calories 353 Fat 14.1g Carbohydrates 44.7g Protein 14g

# Meat and Rotisserie

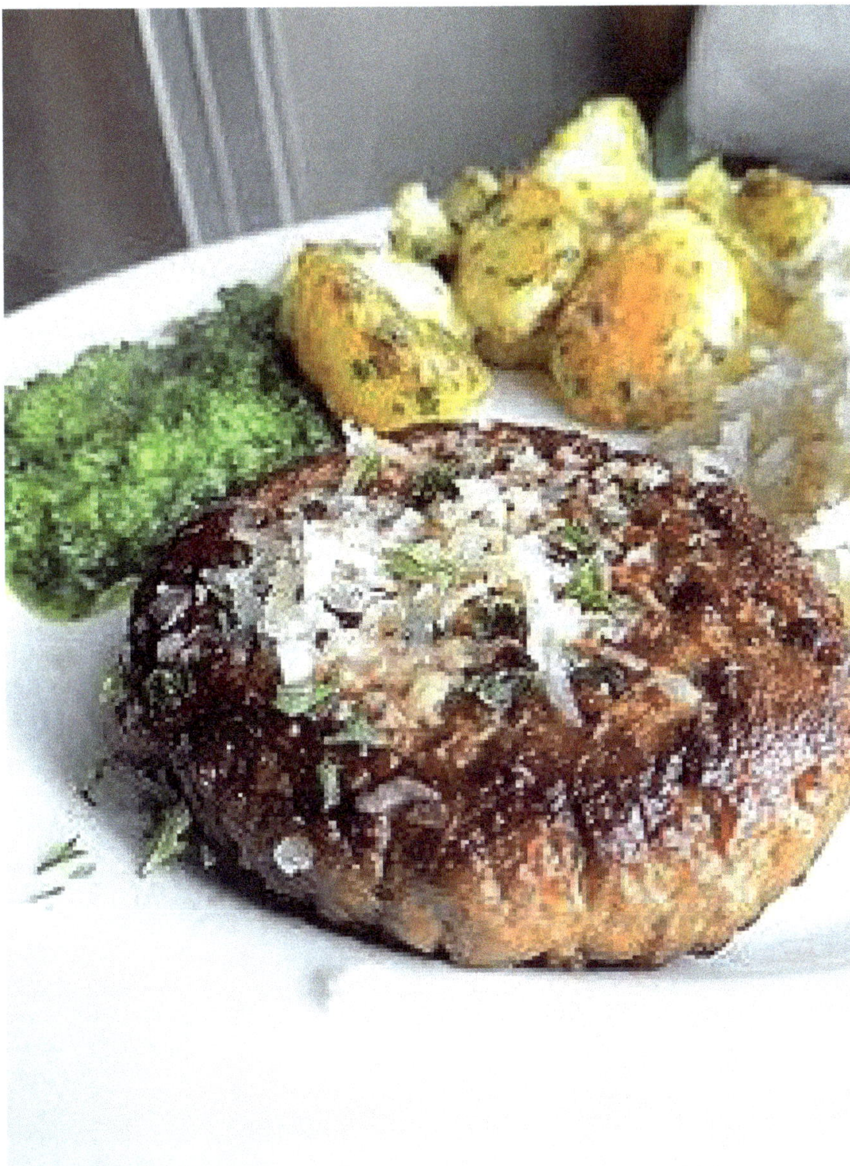

# Blue Cheese Stuffed Burgers

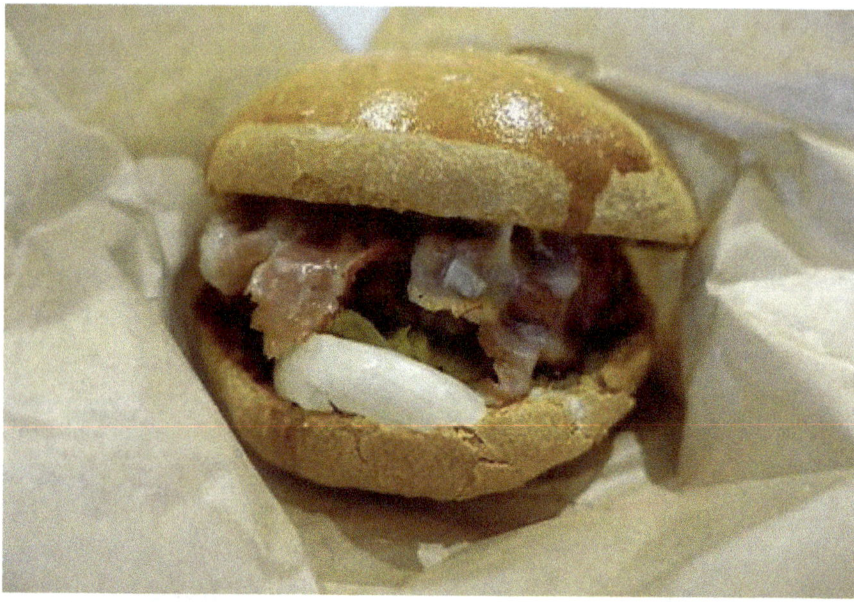

Preparation time: 5 minutes

Cooking time: 22 minutes

Servings: 6

**Ingredients:**

- `2 lb. beef, ground
- `2 tbsp. Worcestershire sauce
- `1 tbsp. salt
- `1/2 tbsp. ground black pepper
- `4 slices of bacon, cooked and chopped
- `8 tbsp. crumbled blue cheese
- `1/4 cup butter
- `4 brioche buns
- `8 slices tomato
- `4 Bibb lettuce leaves
- `4 slices red onion

**Directions:**

1 In a mixing bowl, mix beef, sauce, salt, and pepper until well mixed. Make 4 balls from the mixture then divide each ball into a half.
2 Press the ball on a flat surface. Stuff half of it with bacon and 2 tbsp. cheese. Top with the unstuffed meat and seal the edges.
3 Place the burgers on the air fryer rack.
4 Select the air fry setting of your Kalorik Maxx Air Fryer Oven and set the temperature at 400 degrees Fahrenheit for 18 minutes. Press start.
5 Remove the burgers from the rack and set aside to cool. Transfer the rack to position 1 and butter the buns. Place the buns on the rack, butter side up.
6 Select the broil setting. Set temperature at 400 degrees Fahrenheit for 10 minutes. Broil the buns until golden brown.
7 Assemble the buns and burgers with tomatoes, lettuce leaves, and onions.
8 Serve and enjoy.

**Nutrition:** Calories 590 Carbohydrates 33g Fat 35g Protein 34g

# Air Fried Strip Steak with Red Wine Sauce

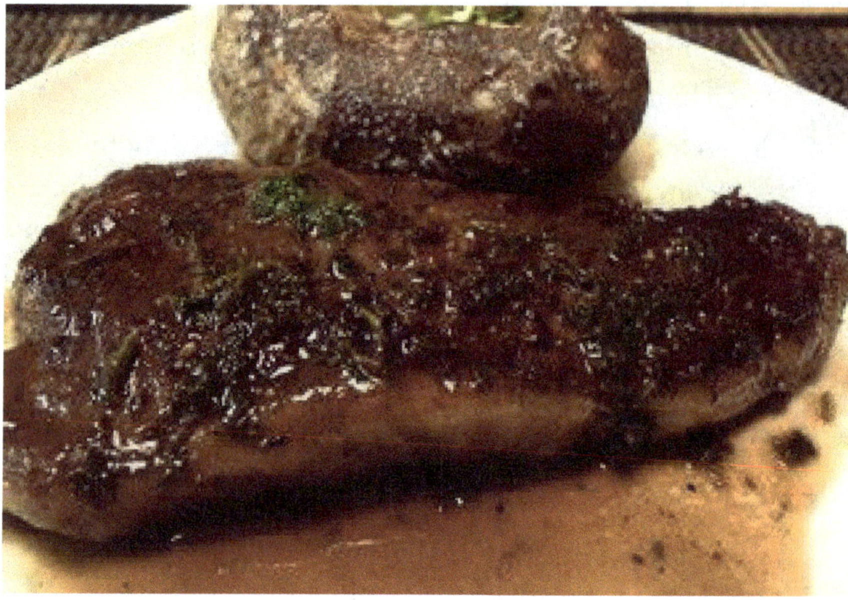

Preparation time: 5 minutes

Cooking time: 20 minutes

Servings: 4

**Ingredients:**

- 1 lb. strip steak, 1 inch thick
- `Salt and pepper
- `1 tbsp. butter, unsalted
- `1/4 cup shallots, chopped
- `1 tbsp. garlic, minced
- `1/2 cup dry red wine
- `2 tbsp. beef bouillon base
- `3 tbsp. heavy cream

**Directions:**

1 Season the steak with salt and pepper and transfer it into the air fryer tray.

2. Select the air fry setting. Set the temperature at 400 degrees Fahrenheit for 10 minutes. When the steak is halfway cooked, turn it so that it can be evenly cooked. Let the steak rest for 10 minutes.
3. Meanwhile, prepare the steak. Melt butter in a saucepan over medium heat. Add shallots, garlic, salt, and pepper. Sauté for 1 minute.
4. Add red wine and bring the mixture to boil. Stir with bouillon base until well mixed. Add heavy cream and cook for 1 more minute.
5. Remove the sauce from heat but keep warm.
6. Slice the steak and serve with the sauce.

**Nutrition:** Calories 649 Carbohydrates 7.5g Fat 34g Protein 69g

# Easy Marinated Steak

Preparation time: 5 minutes

Cooking time: 15 minutes

Servings: 2

**Ingredients:**

- `2 8oz Butcher Box New York strip steaks
- `1 tbsp. soy sauce, low sodium
- `1 tbsp. liquid smoke
- `1 tbsp. McCormick's steak seasoning
- `1/2 tbsp. cocoa powder, unsweetened
- `Salt and pepper to taste
- ` Melted butter

**Directions:**

1 Season the steak with soy sauce and liquid smoke until the steak is well seasoned. Refrigerate for a few hours.

2 Place the steak in the air fryer tray.

3 Select the air fry setting and set the temperature at 370 degrees Fahrenheit for 5 minutes.

4 When the steak is well-cooked, with an internal temperature 160 degrees Fahrenheit, remove from heat and serve it with melted butter. Enjoy.

**Nutrition:** Calories 476 Carbohydrates 1g Fat 28g Protein 49g

## Rib Eye Steak

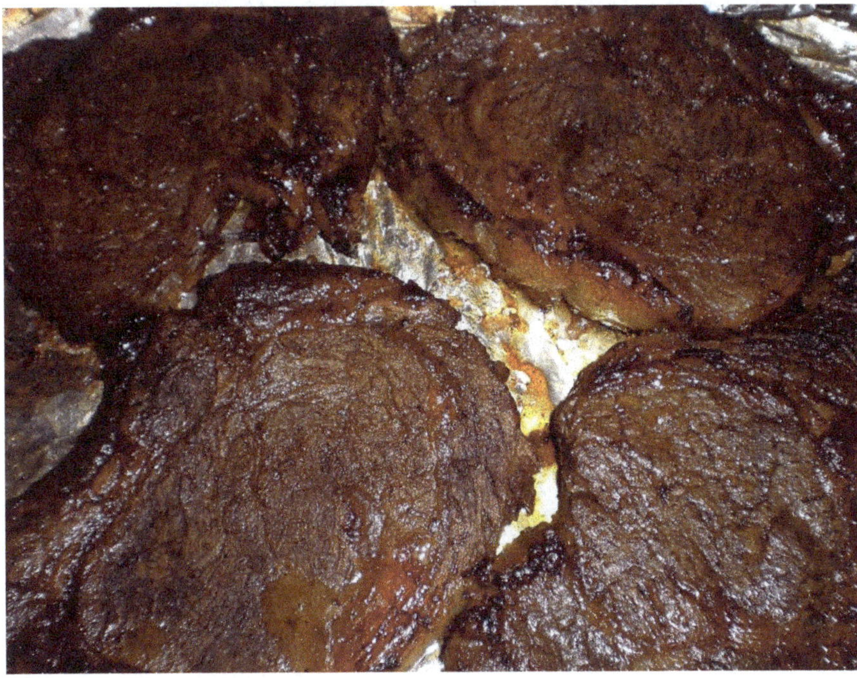

Preparation time: 5 minutes

Cooking time: 22 minutes

Servings: 1

**Ingredients:**

- oz. Rib eye steak
- 1 tbsp. salt
- 3/4 tbsp. pepper
- 1/2 tbsp. garlic powder
- 3/4 steak seasoning

**Directions:**

1 Season the steak with the spices and set aside.

2 Place the steak in the air fryer tray.

3. Select the air fry setting. Set the temperature at 390 degrees Fahrenheit for 12 minutes. Press start.
4. When the steak is halfway cooked, flip it.
5. Transfer the steak to a plate and cover it with a paper foil. Let it rest for 8 minutes before serving it.

**Nutrition:** Calories 651 Carbohydrates 7.5g Fat 49g Protein 44g

## Steak Bites and Mushrooms

Preparation time: 5 minutes

Cooking time: 20 minutes

Servings: 3

**Ingredients:**

- `1 lb. steaks
- `8 oz. mushrooms
- `2 tbsp. butter
- `1 tbsp. Worcestershire sauce
- `1/2 tbsp. garlic powder
- `Salt to taste
- ` Black pepper to taste
- `Minced parsley
- `Melted butter
- `Chili flakes

**Directions:**

1 Pat dry the steak and mushrooms then coat them with butter. Season with Worcestershire sauce, garlic, salt, and pepper.

2 Spread the steak and mushrooms in the air fryer tray.

3 Select the air fry setting of your Kalorik Maxx Air Fryer Oven then set the temperature at 400 degrees Fahrenheit for 18 minutes.

4 Ensure you shake and flip the steak and mushrooms at least 2 times through the cooking process.

5. Garnish with parsley, butter, and chili flakes.
6. Serve when warm.

**Nutrition:** Calories 300 Carbohydrates 2g Fat 21g Protein 24g

## Korean Beef Wraps

Preparation time: 5 minutes

Cooking time: 20 minutes

Servings: 4

**Ingredients:**

- ` 1/4 cup soy sauce, low sodium
- `2 tbsp. orange juice, fresh
- `1 tbsp. dark brown sugar
- `1 tbsp. red pepper flakes
- `1 tbsp. garlic, minced
- `1 bunch scallions, white part
- `2 tbsp. sesame oil
- `1 lb. sirloin steak
- `2 tbsp. sesame seeds, toasted
- `Steamed white rice
- `Kimchi
- `Romaine Lettuce hearts

**Directions:**

1 In a mixing bowl, mix the first 7 ingredients until well combined. Add the steak and toss to coat well.

2 Let the steak stand for at least 4 hours to marinate.

3 Transfer the steak to the air fryer tray.

4 Select the air fry setting of your Kalorik Maxx Air Fryer Oven and set the temperature at 400 degrees Fahrenheit for 10 minutes. Press the start button.

5 When the steak with rice, kimchi wrapped in a lettuce leaf. Enjoy.

**Nutrition:** Calories 298 Carbohydrates 11g Fat 12g Protein 35g

# Hanger Steak with Red wine sauce

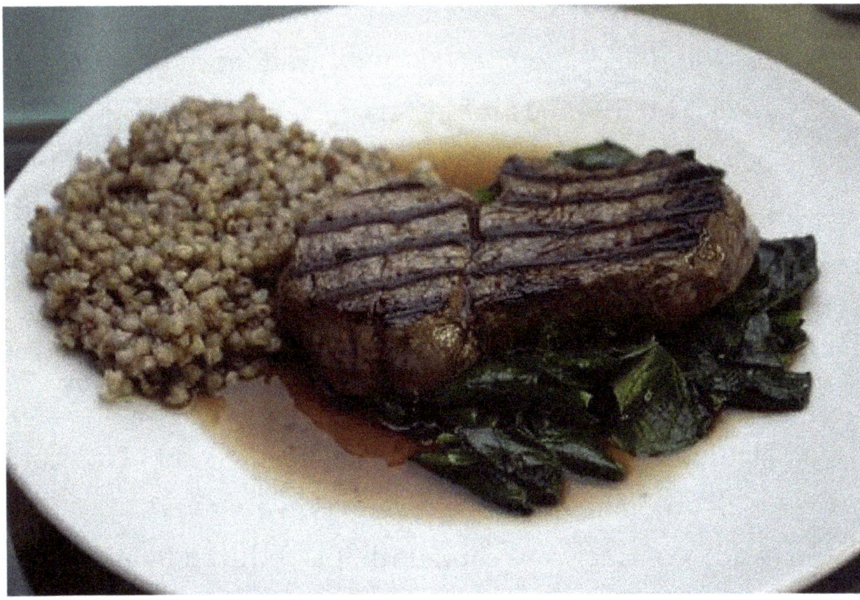

Preparation time: 5 minutes

Cooking time: 25 minutes

Servings: 2

**Ingredients:**

- 7oz hanger steaks
- Salt and pepper
- Oil

For the Sauce

- `1 shallot, thinly sliced
- `2 tbsp. butter
- `1 bottle red wine
- `1 cup bee stock

- `1 tbsp. wholegrain mustard

**Directions:**

1 Season the hanger steak with salt and pepper and transfer it into the air fryer tray.
2 Select the air fry setting on your Kalorik Maxx Air Fryer Oven then set the temperature at 400 degrees Fahrenheit and timer for 10 minutes. When the steak is halfway cooked, turn it so that it can be evenly cooked. Let the steak rest for 10 minutes.
3 Meanwhile, heat a saucepan over medium heat. Cook shallots with butter until translucent. Add wine and cook until almost all the wine has evaporated.
4 Add beef stock and cook until it is reduced by a half.
5 Add mustard and swirl until well combined. Season with salt and pepper to taste.
6 Add a tablespoon of cold butter and swirl the saucepan until it melts. Serve immediately with the hanger steak.

**Nutrition:** Calories 619 Carbohydrates 6.5g Fat 32g Protein 63g

# Air Fried Beef Tenderloin

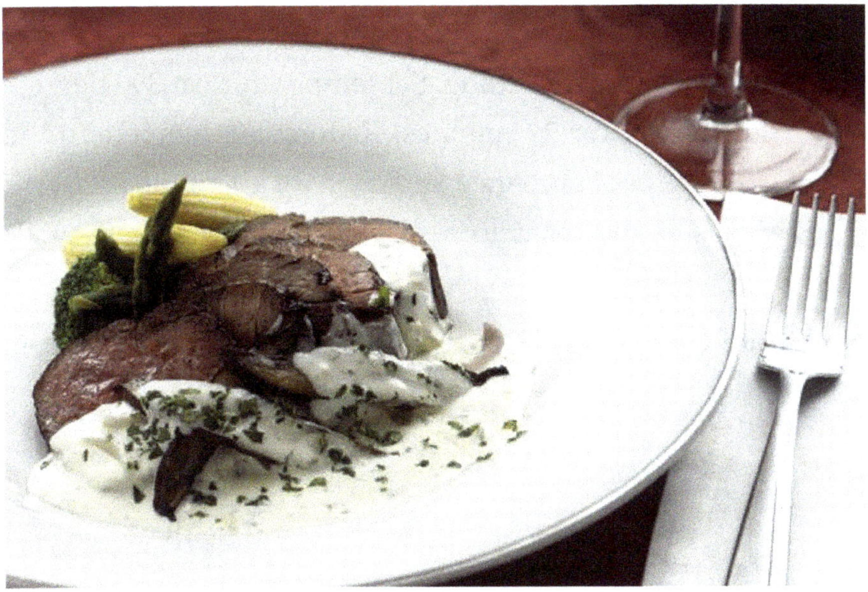

Preparation time: 5 minutes

Cooking time: 47 minutes

Servings: 8

**Ingredients:**

- `2 lb. beef tenderloin
- `1 tbsp. vegetable oil
- `1 tbsp. dried oregano
- `1 tbsp. salt
- `1/2 tbsp. black pepper, cracked

**Directions:**

1 Pat dry the tenderloin with a paper towel and place it on a platter.

2. Drizzle vegetable oil and sprinkle oregano, salt, and pepper. Rub the spices on the meat until well coated.
3. Place the roast on the air fryer tray.
4. Select the air fry setting. Set temperature at 390 degrees Fahrenheit for 22 minutes. Reduce the temperature to 360 degrees Fahrenheit and cook for 10 minutes.
5. Transfer the meat to a plate and allow to rest while tented with paper foil for 10 minutes before serving.

**Nutrition:** Calories 235 Carbohydrates 0.2g Fat 10.6g Protein 32.4g

# Poultry

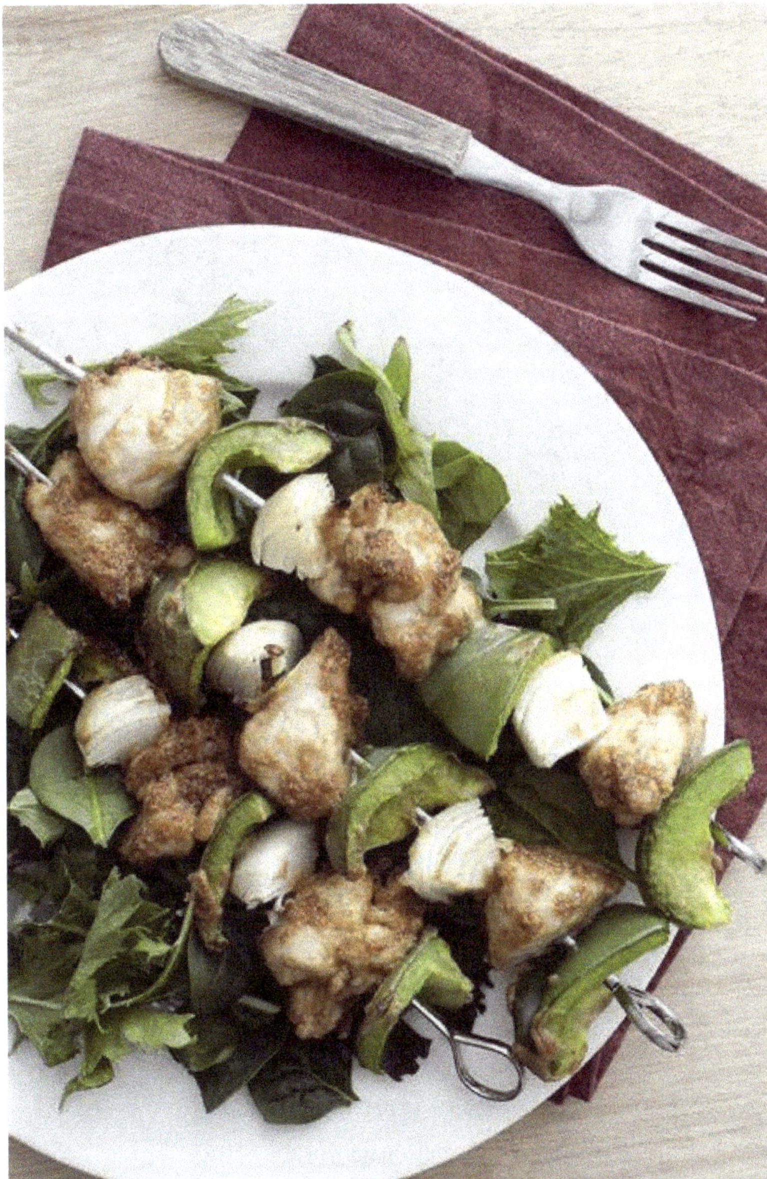

## Chicken Parm

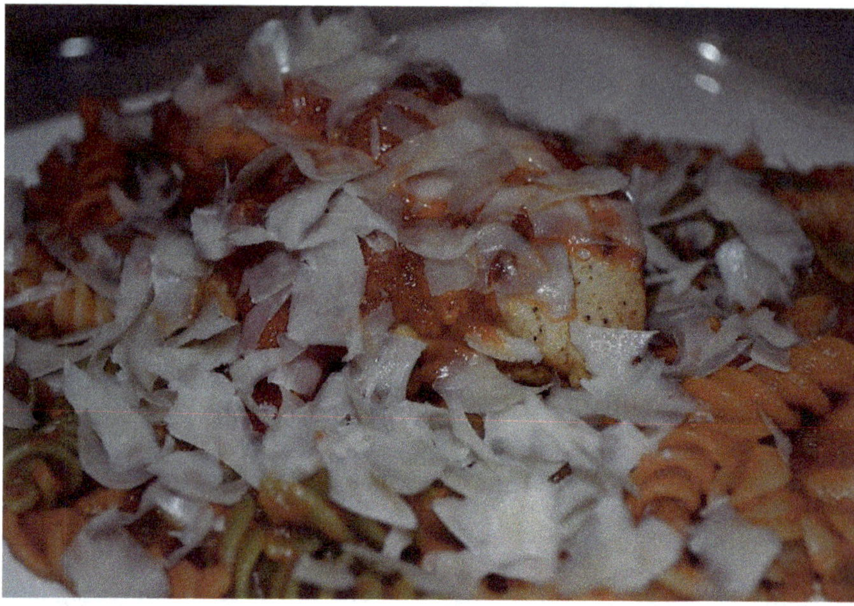

Preparation Time: 10 minutes

Cooking time: 35 minutes

Servings: 4

**Ingredients:**

- Nonstick cooking spray
- ½ cup flour
- 2 eggs
- 2/3 cup panko bread crumbs
- 2/3 cup Italian seasoned bread crumbs
- 1/3 + ¼ cup parmesan cheese, divided
- 2 tbsp. fresh parsley, chopped
- ½ tsp salt
- ¼ tsp pepper

- 4 chicken breast halves, skinless and boneless
- 24 oz. marinara sauce
- 1 cup mozzarella cheese, grated

**Directions**

1. Place the baking pan in position 2 of the oven. Lightly spray the fryer basket with cooking spray.
2. Place flour in a shallow dish.
3. In a separate shallow dish, beat the eggs.
4. In a third shallow dish, combine both bread crumbs, 1/3 cup parmesan cheese, 2 tablespoons parsley, salt, and pepper.
5. Place chicken between two sheets of plastic wrap and pound to ½-inch thick.
6. Dip chicken first in flour, then eggs, and bread crumb mixture to coat. Place in basket and place the basket on the baking pan.
7. Set oven to air fry on 375 degrees Fahrenheit for 10 minutes. Turn chicken over halfway through cooking time.
8. Remove chicken and baking pan from the oven. Place the rack in position 1. Set oven to bake on 425 degrees Fahrenheit for 30 minutes.
9. Pour 1 ½ cups marinara in the bottom of 8x11-inch baking dish. Place chicken over sauce and add another 2 tablespoons marinara to tops of chicken. Top chicken with mozzarella and parmesan cheese

10. Once oven preheats for 5 minutes, place the dish in the oven and bake 20-25 minutes until bubbly and cheese is golden brown. Serve.

**Nutrition:** Calories 529 Total Fat 13g Saturated Fat 5g Cholesterol 0mg Sodium 1437mg Total Carbohydrate 52g Fiber 5g Sugar 9g Protein 51g

## Teriyaki Duck Legs

Preparation Time: 15 minutes

Cooking time: 2 hours

Servings: 6

**Ingredients:**

- 3 lbs. duck legs
- ½ cup teriyaki sauce
- 2 tbsp. soy sauce
- 2 tbsp. malt vinegar

**Directions**

1. Place the rack in position 1 of the oven.
2. Place the duck legs, skin side up, in an 8x11-inch baking dish.
3. In a small bowl, whisk together remaining ingredients and pour around duck legs. Liquid needs to reach the skin level of duck, if not add water until it does.
4. Set the oven to convection bake on 300 degrees Fahrenheit for 60 minutes. After 5 minutes, place the ducks in the oven and cook 90 minutes, or until tender.
5. Remove duck from the oven. Pour off cooking liquid into a small saucepan. Skim off fat and reserve. Bring sauce to a boil and cook until it reduces down, about 10 minutes, stirring occasionally.
6. Place the baking pan in position 2 of the oven. Place the duck legs in the fryer basket and brush with reserved fat

and sauce. Place the basket in the oven and set to broil on 400 degrees Fahrenheit for 10 minutes. Turn duck over halfway through and brush with fat and sauce again. Serve.

**Nutrition:** Calories 608 Total Fat 20g Saturated Fat 5g Cholesterol 0mg Sodium 1063mg Total Carbohydrate 6g Fiber 0g Sugar 5g Protein 101g

## Almond Flour Coco-Milk Battered Chicken

Preparation Time: 5 minutes

Cooking time: 30 minutes

Servings: 4

**Ingredients:**

- ¼ cup coconut milk
- ½ cup almond flour
- 1 ½ tablespoons old bay Cajun seasoning
- 1 egg, beaten
- 4 small chicken thighs
- Salt and pepper to taste

**Directions**

1. Preheat the air fryer oven for 5 minutes.
2. Mix the egg and coconut milk in a bowl.
3. Soak the chicken thighs in the beaten egg mixture.
4. In a mixing bowl, combine the almond flour, Cajun seasoning, salt and pepper.
5. Dredge the chicken thighs in the almond flour mixture.
6. Place in the air fryer basket.
7. Cook for 30 minutes at 350 degrees Fahrenheit.

**Nutrition:** Calories 590 Total Fat 38g Saturated Fat 0g Cholesterol 0mg Sodium 0mg Total Carbohydrate 3.2g Fiber 0g Sugar 0g Protein 32.5g

## Sweet and Sour Chicken

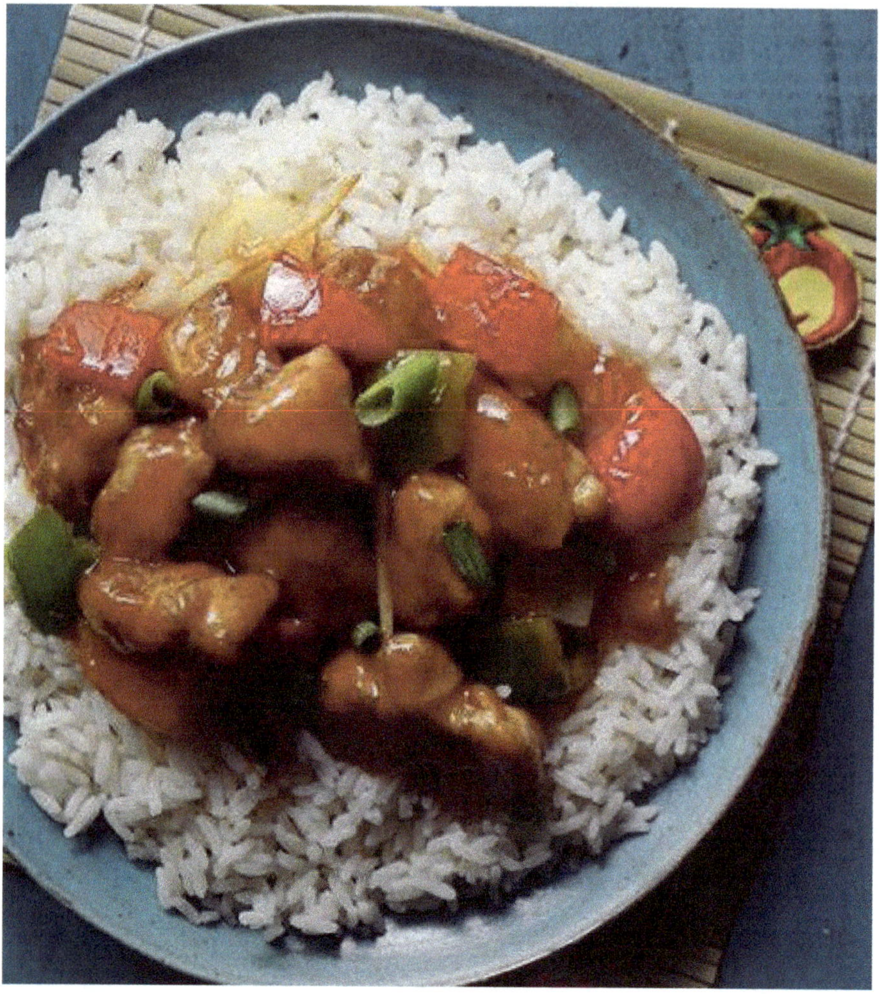

Preparation Time: 5 minutes

Cooking time: 20 minutes

Servings: 6

**Ingredients:**

- 3 Chicken Breasts, cubed
- 1/2 Cup Flour
- 1/2 Cup Cornstarch
- 2 Red Peppers, sliced
- 1 Onion, chopped
- 2 Carrots, julienned
- 3/4 Cup Sugar
- 2 Tbsps Cornstarch
- 1/3 Cup Vinegar
- 2/3 Cup Water
- 1/4 cup Soy sauce
- 1 Tbsp Ketchup

**Directions**

1. Preheat the air fryer oven to 375 degrees Fahrenheit.
2. Combine the flour, cornstarch and chicken in an air tight container and shake to combine
3. Remove chicken from the container and shake off any excess flour.
4. Add chicken to the Air Fryer tray and cook for 20 minutes.
5. In a saucepan, whisk together sugar, water, vinegar, soy sauce and ketchup. Bring to a boil over medium heat, reduce the heat then simmer for 2 minutes
6. After cooking the chicken for 20 minutes, add the vegetables and sauce mixture to the air fryer oven and cook for another 5 minutes
7. Serve over hot rice

**Nutrition:** Calories 300 Total Fat 0g Saturated Fat 0g Cholesterol 0mg Sodium 260mg Total Carbohydrate 40g Fiber 1g Sugar 24g Protein 0g

# Fish and Seafood

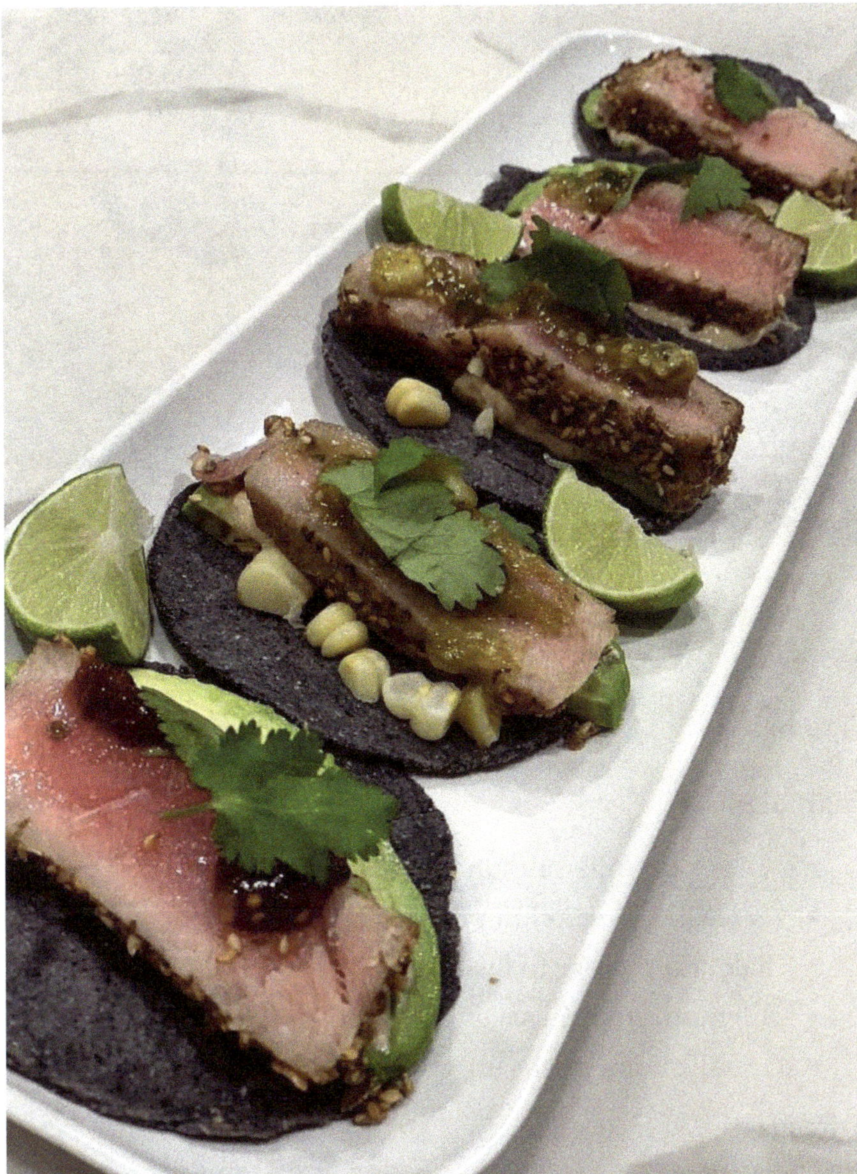

## Lemon Salmon

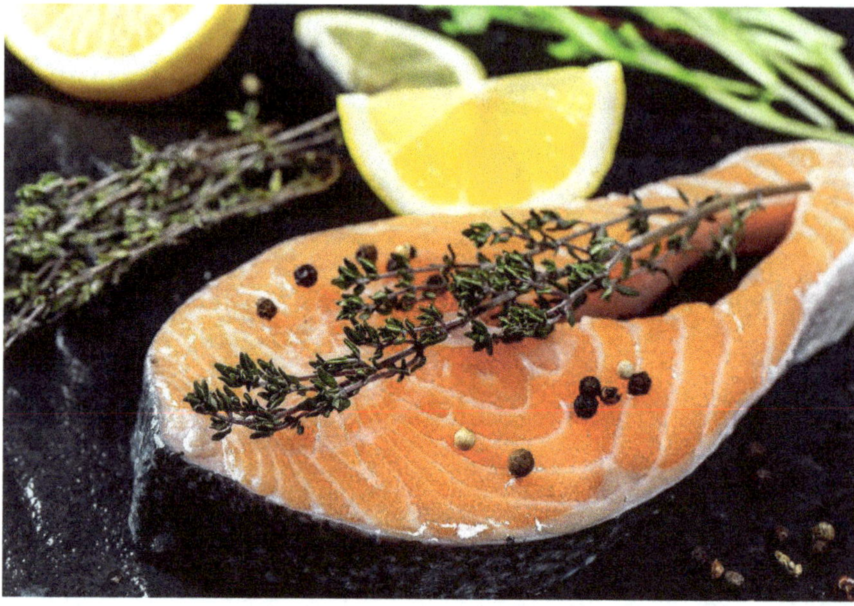

Preparation Time: 10 minutes

Cooking Time: 8 minutes

Servings: 3

**Ingredients:**

- and ½ pounds salmon
- ½ teaspoon red chili powder
- Salt and pepper to taste
- 1 lemon, cut into slices
- 1 tablespoon fresh dill, chopped

**Directions:**

1 Season salmon with chili powder, salt, pepper generously

2. Press "Power Button" on your Air Fryer and select "Air Fry" mode
3. Press the Time Button and set time to 8 minutes
4. Push Temp Button and set temp to 375 degrees F
5. Press the "Start/Pause" button and start the device
6. Once the appliance beeps to indicated that it is pre-heated, arrange salmon fillets in the Air Fryer cooking basket
7. Push into Air Fryer Oven and cook until the timer runs out
8. Garnish with fresh dill and serve hot!

**Nutrition:** Calories: 305 Fat: 14 g Saturated Fat: 2 g Carbohydrates: 1.3 g Fiber: 0.4 g Sodium: 156 mg Protein: 44 g

## Hearty Spiced Salmon

Preparation Time: 10 minutes

Cooking Time: 11 minutes

Servings: 2

**Ingredients:**

- teaspoon smoked paprika
- 1 teaspoon cayenne pepper
- 1 teaspoon onion powder
- 1 teaspoon garlic powder
- Salt and pepper to taste
- pieces 6 ounces salmon fillets
- teaspoons olive oil

**Directions:**

1 Take a small bowl and add spices, mix them well

2 Drizzle salmon fillets with oil, rub the fillets with spice mixture

3 Press "Power Button" on your Air Fryer and select "Air Fry" mode

4 Press the Time Button and set time to 11 minutes

5 Push Temp Button and set temp to 390 degrees F

6 Press the "Start/Pause" button and start the device

7 Once the appliance beeps to indicated that it is pre-heated, arrange salmon fillets in the Air Fryer cooking basket

8. Push into Air Fryer Oven and cook until the timer runs out
9. Serve and enjoy!

**Nutrition:** Calories: 280 Fat: 15 g Saturated Fat: 2 g Carbohydrates: 3 g Fiber: 1 g Sodium: 0.8 mg Protein: 33 g

## Cajun Shrimp

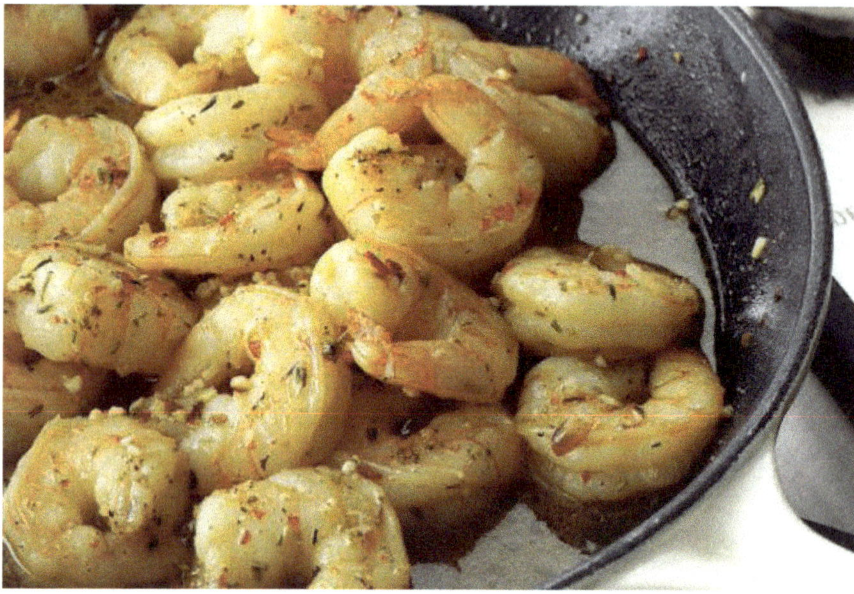

Preparation Time: 10 minutes

Cooking Time: 7 minutes

Servings: 4

**Ingredients:**

- and ¼ pound tiger shrimp, about 16-20 pieces
- ¼ teaspoon cayenne pepper
- ½ teaspoon old bay seasoning
- ¼ teaspoon smoked paprika
- 1 pinch of salt
- 1 tablespoon olive oil

**Directions:**

1. Preheat your Air Fryer to 390 degrees F in "AIR FRY" mode
2. Take a mixing bowl and add ingredients (except shrimp), mix well
3. Dip the shrimp into spice mixture and oil
4. Transfer the prepared shrimp to your cooking basket and cook for 5 minutes
5. Serve and enjoy!

**Nutrition:** Calories: 180 Fat: 2 g Saturated Fat: 1 g Carbohydrates: 5 g Fiber: 0 g Sodium: 970 mg Protein: 23 g

## Air Fried Dragon Shrimp

Preparation Time: 10 minutes

Cooking Time: 10 minutes

Servings: 4

**Ingredients:**

- 1-pound raw shrimp, peeled and deveined
- A ½ cup of soy sauce
- eggs
- tablespoons olive oil
- cup yellow onion, diced
- ¼ cup flour
- ½ teaspoon red pepper, ground
- ½ teaspoon ginger, grounded

**Directions:**

1 Preheat your air fryer to 350 degrees F in "AIR FRY" mode
2 Add all the ingredients except for the shrimp to make the batter
3 Set it aside for 10 minutes
4 Dip each shrimp into the batter to coat all sides
5 Place them on the air fryer basket
6 Cook for 10 minutes
7 Serve and enjoy!

**Nutrition:** Calories: 600 Fat: 6 g Saturated Fat: 2 g Carbohydrates: 59 g Fiber: 8 g Sodium: 690 mg Protein: 31 g

## Mushroom And Tilapia

Preparation Time: 10 minutes

Cooking Time: 16 minutes

Servings: 4

**Ingredients:**

- ½ cup yellow onion, sliced thin
- ounces filets tilapia
- tablespoons olive oil
- cups mushroom, sliced
- tablespoons soy sauce
- cloves garlic, minced
- tablespoon honey
- tablespoons rice vinegar
- and ½ teaspoon salt
- 1 tablespoon red chili flakes

**Directions:**

1 Preheat your air fryer to 350 degrees F in "AIR FRY" mode
2 Season the fish with half the salt
3 Drizzle with half the oil
4 Cook for 15 minutes
5 Take a large skillet and add remaining oil and heat it
6 Add the onion, garlic, and mushroom when it is hot
7 Cook until onions are soft
8 Stir in the soy sauce, honey, vinegar, and chili flakes

9. Simmer for 1 minute
10. Serve with mushroom sauce and enjoy!

**Nutrition:** Calories: 300 Fat: 10 g Saturated Fat: 2 g Carbohydrates: 12 g Fiber: 4 g Sodium: 609 mg Protein: 45 g

# Bacon-Wrapped Shrimp

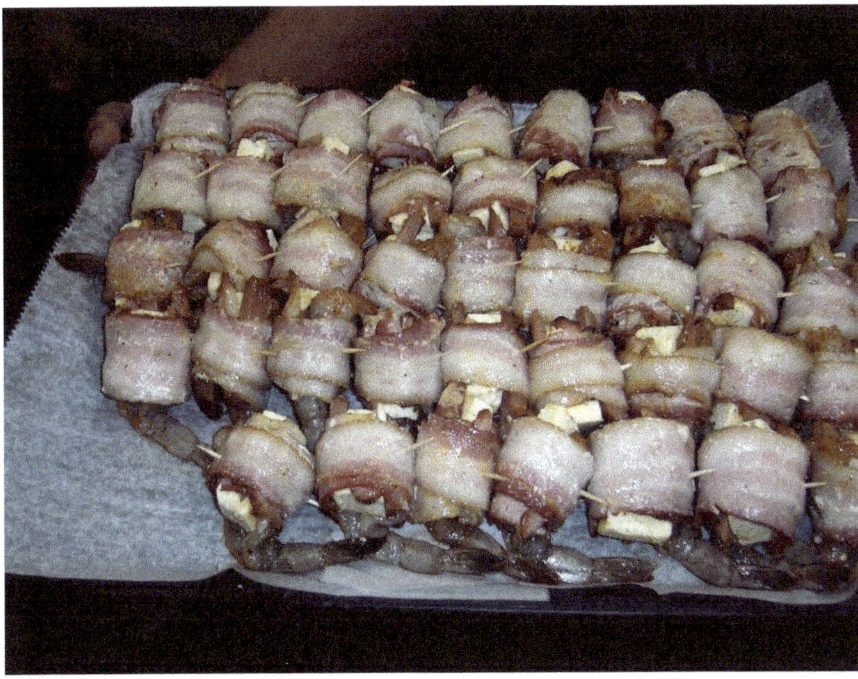

Preparation time: 5 minutes

Cooking time: 5 minutes

Servings: 4

**Ingredients**

- 1¼ pound tiger shrimp, peeled and deveined
- pound bacon

**Directions:**

1 Preparing the Ingredients. Wrap each shrimp with a slice of bacon.
2 Refrigerate for about 20 minutes.
3 Preheat the Air fryer oven to 390 degrees F.

4. Air Frying. Arrange the shrimp in the Oven rack/basket. Place the Rack on the middle-shelf of the Air fryer oven. Cook for about 5-7 minutes.

**Nutrition:** Calories 70 Total Fat 4.5g Total Carbs 0g Fiber 0g Protein 7g Sugar 0g Sodium 150mg

# Baking

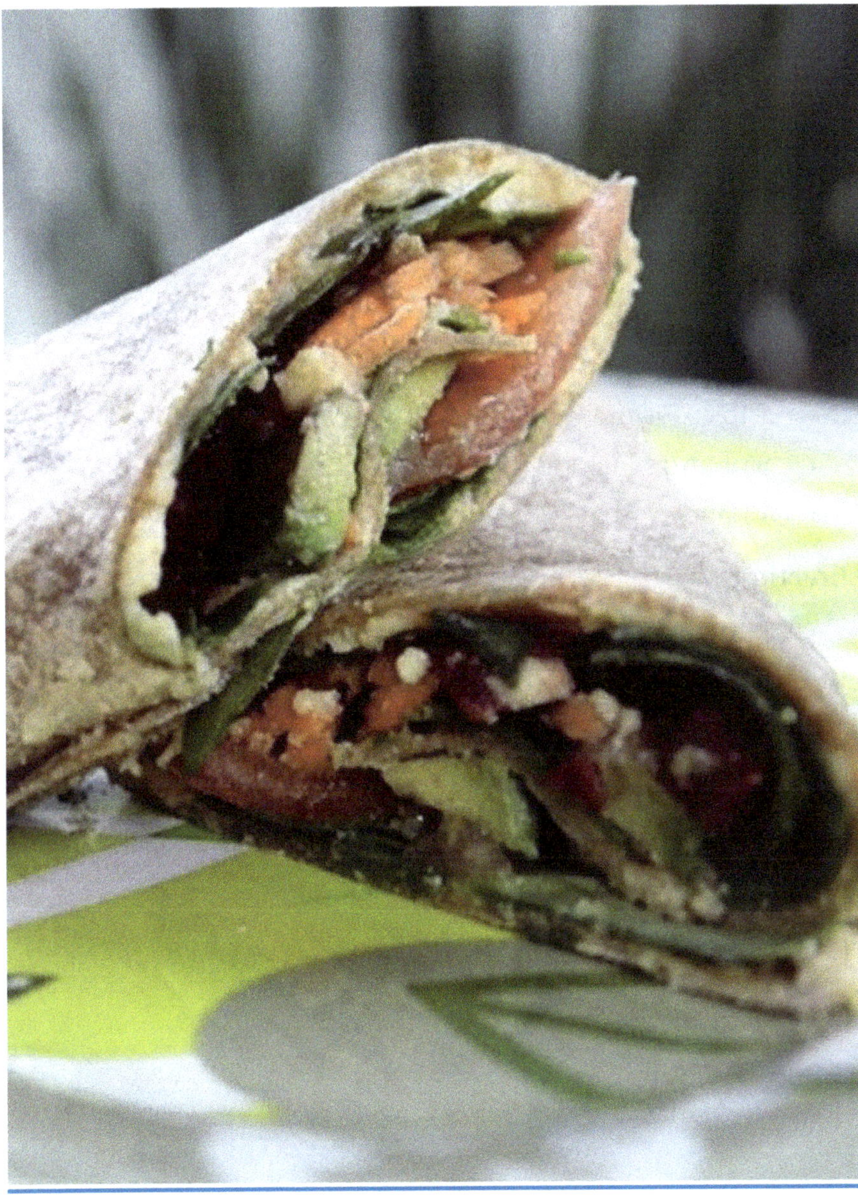

## Basil Parmesan Bagel

Preparation time: 5 minutes

Cooking time: 10 minutes

Servings: 1

**Ingredients:**

- 2 tbsp butter, softened
- ¼ tsp dried basil
- 1 tsp garlic powder
- 1 tbsp Parmesan cheese, grated
- Salt and black pepper to taste
- 1 bagel

**Directions**

1 Preheat on Bake function to 370 degrees Fahrenheir. Cut the bagel in half. Combine the butter, Parmesan cheese, garlic, and basil in a small bowl. Season with salt and pepper. Spread the mixture onto the halved bagel. Place the bagel in the basket and press Start. Cook for 5-6 minutes.

**Nutrition:** Calories 131 Fat 0g Carbohydrates 27g Proteins 5g

## Buttery Orange Toasts

Preparation time: 5 minutes

Cooking time: 10 minutes

Servings: 6

**Ingredients:**

- 12 bread slices
- ½ cup sugar
- 1 stick butter
- 1 ½ tbsp vanilla extract
- 1 ½ tbsp cinnamon
- 2 oranges, zested

**Directions**

1 Mix butter, sugar, and vanilla extract and microwave the mixture for 30 seconds until it melts. Add in orange zest. Spread the mixture onto bread slices. Lay the bread slices on the cooking basket and cook in the oven for 5 minutes at 400 degrees Fahrenheit on Toast function. Serve warm.

**Nutrition:** Calories 131 Fat 0g Carbohydrates 27g Proteins 5g

# Basil Prosciutto Crostini with Mozzarella

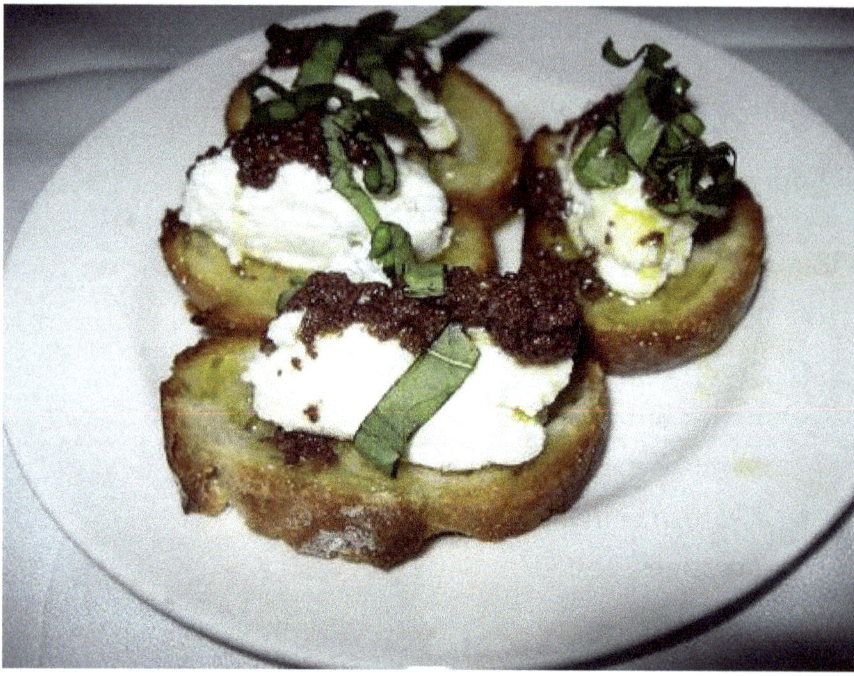

Preparation time: 5 minutes

Cooking time: 10 minutes

Servings: 1

**Ingredients:**

- ½ cup tomatoes, chopped
- 3 oz mozzarella cheese, chopped
- 3 prosciutto slices, chopped
- 1 tbsp olive oil
- 1 tsp dried basil
- 6 small slices of French bread

**Preparation**

1. Preheat on Toast function to 350 degrees F. Place in the bread slices and toast them for 5 minutes. Top the bread with tomatoes, prosciutto, and mozzarella. Sprinkle with basil. Drizzle with olive oil. Return to oven and cook for 1 more minute, enough to become melty and warm.

**Nutrition:** Calories 411 Fat 23g Carbohydrates 41g Proteins 16g

# Soda Bread

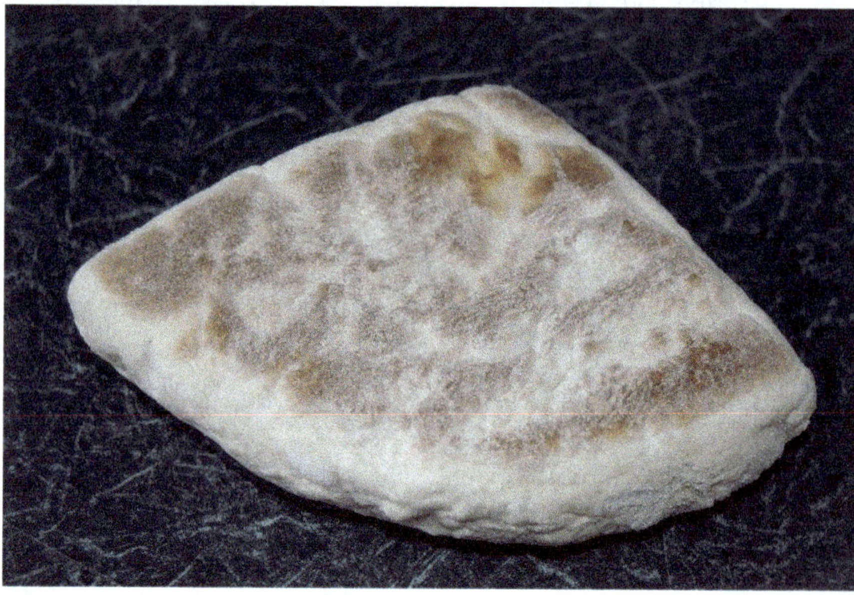

Preparation Time: 15 minutes

Cooking time: 30 minutes

Servings: 10

**Ingredients:**

- 3 cups whole-wheat flour
- 1 tablespoon sugar
- 2 teaspoon caraway seeds
- 1 teaspoon baking soda
- 1 teaspoon sea salt
- ¼ cup chilled butter, cubed into small pieces
- 1 large egg, beaten
- 1½ cups buttermilk

**Directions**

1. In a large bowl, mix together the flour, sugar, caraway seeds, baking soda and salt and mix well.
2. With a pastry cutter, cut in the butter flour until coarse crumbs like mixture is formed.
3. Make a well in the center of flour mixture.
4. In the well, add the egg, followed by the buttermilk and with a spatula, mix until well combined.
5. With floured hand, shape the dough into a ball.
6. Place the dough onto a floured surface and lightly knead it.
7. Shape the dough into a 6-inch ball.
8. With a serrated knife, score an X on the top of the dough.
9. Press "Power Button" of Air Fry Oven and turn the dial to select the "Air Crisp" mode.
10. Press the Time button and again turn the dial to set the cooking time to 30 minutes.
11. Now push the Temp button and rotate the dial to set the temperature at 350 degrees Fahrenheit.
12. Press "Start/Pause" button to start.
13. When the unit beeps to show that it is preheated, open the lid.
14. Arrange the dough in lightly greased "Air Fry Basket" and insert in the oven.
15. Place the pan onto a wire rack to cool for about 10 minutes.
16. Carefully, invert the bread onto wire rack to cool completely before slicing.

17 Cut the bread into desired-sized slices and serve.

**Nutrition:** Calories 205 Total Fat 5.9g Saturated Fat 3.3g Cholesterol 32mg Sodium 392mg Total Carbohydrates 31.8g Fiber 1.2g Sugar 3.1g Protein 5.9g

# Baguette Bread

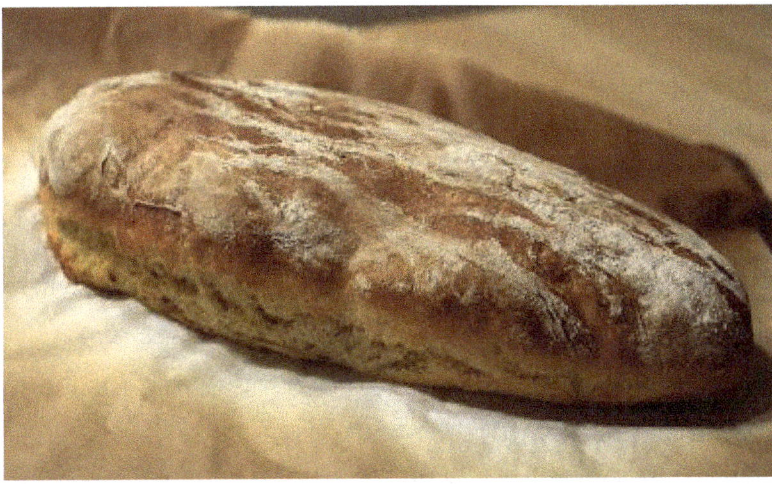

Preparation Time: 15 minutes

Cooking time: 20 minutes

Servings: 8

**Ingredients:**

- ¾ cup warm water
- ¾ teaspoon quick yeast
- ½ teaspoon demerara sugar
- 1 cup bread flour
- ½ cup whole-wheat flour
- ½ cup oat flour
- 1¼ teaspoons salt

**Directions**

1 In a large bowl, place the water and sprinkle with yeast and sugar.

2 Set aside for 5 minutes or until foamy.

3. Add the bread flour and salt mix until a stiff dough forms.
4. Put the dough onto a floured surface and with your hands, knead until smooth and elastic.
5. Now, shape the dough into a ball.
6. Place the dough into a slightly oiled bowl and turn to coat well.
7. With a plastic wrap, cover the bowl and place in a warm place for about 1 hour or until doubled in size.
8. With your hands, punch down the dough and form into a long slender loaf.
9. Place the loaf onto a lightly greased baking sheet and set aside in warm place, uncovered, for about 30 minutes.
10. Press "Power Button" of Air Fry Oven and turn the dial to select the "Air Bake" mode.
11. Press the Time button and again turn the dial to set the cooking time to 20 minutes.
12. Now push the Temp button and rotate the dial to set the temperature at 450 degrees Fahrenheit.
13. Press "Start/Pause" button to start.
14. When the unit beeps to show that it is preheated, open the lid.
15. Carefully, arrange the dough onto the "Wire Rack" and insert in the oven.
16. Carefully, invert the bread onto wire rack to cool completely before slicing.
17. Cut the bread into desired-sized slices and serve.

**Nutrition:** Calories 114 Total Fat 0.8g Saturated Fat 0.1g Cholesterol 0mg Sodium 366mg Total Carbohydrates 22.8g Fiber 2.1g Sugar 0.3g Protein 3.8g

# Yogurt Bread

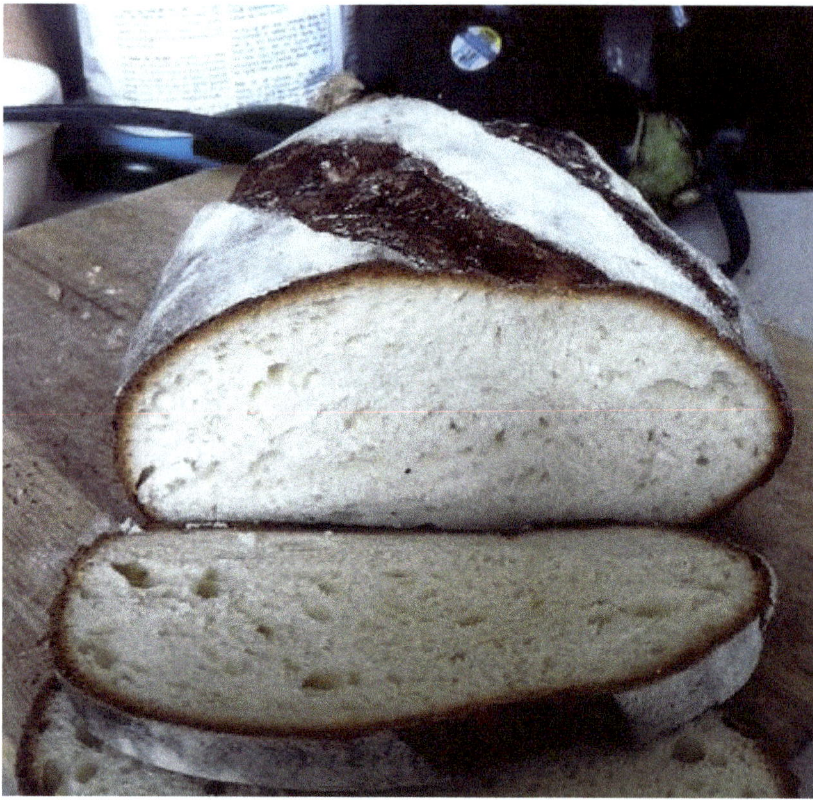

Preparation Time: 20 minutes

Cooking time: 40 minutes

Servings: 10

**Ingredients:**

- 1½ cups warm water, divided
- 1½ teaspoons active dry yeast
- 1 teaspoon sugar
- 3 cups all-purpose flour

- 1 cup plain Greek yogurt
- 2 teaspoons kosher salt

**Directions**

1 Add ½ cup of the warm water, yeast and sugar in the bowl of a stand mixer, fitted with the dough hook attachment and mix well.
2 Set aside for about 5 minutes.
3 Add the flour, yogurt, and salt and mix on medium-low speed until the dough comes together.
4 Then, mix on medium speed for 5 minutes.
5 Place the dough into a bowl.
6 With a plastic wrap, cover the bowl and place in a warm place for about 2-3 hours or until doubled in size.
7 Transfer the dough onto a lightly floured surface and shape into a smooth ball.
8 Place the dough onto a greased parchment paper-lined rack.
9 With a kitchen towel, cover the dough and let rest for 15 minutes.
10 With a very sharp knife, cut a 4x½-inch deep cut down the center of the dough.
11 Press "Power Button" of Air Fry Oven and turn the dial to select the "Air Roast" mode.
12 Press the Time button and again turn the dial to set the cooking time to 40 minutes.
13 Now push the Temp button and rotate the dial to set the temperature at 325 degrees Fahrenheit.
14 Press "Start/Pause" button to start.

15 When the unit beeps to show that it is preheated, open the lid.
16 Carefully, arrange the dough onto the "Wire Rack" and insert in the oven.
17 Carefully, invert the bread onto wire rack to cool completely before slicing.
18 Cut the bread into desired-sized slices and serve.

**Nutrition:** Calories 157 Total Fat 0.7g Saturated Fat 0.3g Cholesterol 1mg Sodium 484mg Total Carbohydrates 31g Fiber 1.1g Sugar 2.2g Protein 5.5g

# Measurement Conversion Chart

| American and British Variances | | | | | |
|---|---|---|---|---|---|
| **Term** | **Abbreviation** | **Nationality** | **Dry or liquid** | **Metric equivalent** | **Equivalent in context** |
| **cup** | c., C. | | usually liquid | 237 milliliters | 16 tablespoons or 8 ounces |
| **ounce** | fl oz, fl. oz. | American | liquid only | 29.57 milliliters | |
| | | British | either | 28.41 milliliters | |
| **gallon** | gal. | American | liquid only | 3.785 liters | 4 quarts |
| | | British | either | 4.546 liters | 4 quarts |
| **inch** | in, in. | | | 2.54 centimeters | |
| **ounce** | oz, oz. | American | dry | 28.35 grams | 1/16 pound |
| | | | liquid | see OUNCE | see OUNCE |
| **pint** | p., pt. | American | liquid | 0.473 liter | 1/8 gallon or 16 ounces |
| | | | dry | 0.551 liter | 1/2 quart |
| | | British | either | 0.568 liter | |
| **pound** | lb. | | dry | 453.592 grams | 16 ounces |
| **Quart** | q., qt, qt. | American | liquid | 0.946 liter | 1/4 gallon or 32 ounces |
| | | | dry | 1.101 liters | 2 pints |
| | | British | either | 1.136 liters | |
| **Teaspoon** | t., tsp., tsp | | either | about 5 milliliters | 1/3 tablespoon |
| **Tablespoon** | T., tbs., tbsp. | | either | about 15 milliliters | 3 teaspoons or 1/2 ounce |

## Volume (Liquid)

| American Standard (Cups & Quarts ) | American Standard (Ounces) | Metric (Milliliters & Liters) |
|---|---|---|
| 2 tbsp. | 1 fl. oz. | 30 ml |
| 1/4 cup | 2 fl. oz. | 60 ml |
| 1/2 cup | 4 fl. oz. | 125 ml |
| 1 cup | 8 fl. oz. | 250 ml |
| 1 1/2 cups | 12 fl. oz. | 375 ml |
| 2 cups or 1 pint | 16 fl. oz. | 500 ml |
| 4 cups or 1 quart | 32 fl. oz. | 1000 ml or 1 liter |
| 1 gallon | 128 fl. oz. | 4 liters |

## Volume (Dry)

| American Standard | Metric |
|---|---|
| 1/8 teaspoon | 5 ml |
| 1/4 teaspoon | 1 ml |
| 1/2 teaspoon | 2 ml |
| 3/4 teaspoon | 4 ml |
| 1 teaspoon | 5 ml |
| 1 tablespoon | 15 ml |
| 1/4 cup | 59 ml |
| 1/3 cup | 79 ml |
| 1/2 cup | 118 ml |
| 2/3 cup | 158 ml |
| 3/4 cup | 177 ml |
| 1 cup | 225 ml |
| 2 cups or 1 pint | 450 ml |
| 3 cups | 675 ml |
| 4 cups or 1 quart | 1 liter |
| 1/2 gallon | 2 liters |
| 1 gallon | 4 liters |

## Dry Measure Equivalents

| | | | |
|---|---|---|---|
| 3 teaspoons | 1 tablespoon | 1/2 ounce | 14.3 grams |
| 2 tablespoons | 1/8 cup | 1 ounce | 28.3 grams |
| 4 tablespoons | 1/4 cup | 2 ounces | 56.7 grams |
| 5 1/3 tablespoons | 1/3 cup | 2.6 ounces | 75.6 grams |
| 8 tablespoons | 1/2 cup | 4 ounces | 113.4 grams |
| 12 tablespoons | 3/4 cup | 6 ounces | .375 pound |
| 32 tablespoons | 2 cups | 16 ounces | 1 pound |

## Oven Temperatures

| American Standard | Metric |
|---|---|
| 250° F | 130° C |
| 300° F | 150° C |
| 350° F | 180° C |
| 400° F | 200° C |
| 450° F | 230° C |

## Weight (Mass)

| American Standard (Ounces) | Metric (Grams) |
|---|---|
| 1/2 ounce | 15 grams |
| 1 ounce | 30 grams |
| 3 ounces | 85 grams |
| 3.75 ounces | 100 grams |
| 4 ounces | 115 grams |
| 8 ounces | 225 grams |
| 12 ounces | 340 grams |
| 16 ounces or 1 pound | 450 grams |

CPSIA information can be obtained
at www.ICGtesting.com
Printed in the USA
LVHW080747090621
689715LV00006B/263

9 781803 111452